A Study Guide to Epidemiology and Biostatistics

Second Edition

A Study Guide to Epidemiology and Biostatistics
including 100 multiple-choice questions

Second Edition

**Richard F. Morton,
M.B.B.S., M.P.H., F.A.C.P.M.,
F.A.C.E.**

*Associate Clinical Professor
Department of Community Health
Albert Einstein College of Medicine
Yeshiva University
New York, New York,
Associate Director for Medical Services
March of Dimes–Birth Defects Foundation
White Plains, New York*

J. Richard Hebel, Ph.D.

*Associate Professor
Department of Epidemiology and Preventive Medicine
University of Maryland School of Medicine
Baltimore, Maryland*

University Park Press . Baltimore

University Park Press
International Publishers in Medicine and Allied Health
300 North Charles Street
Baltimore, Maryland 21201

Sponsoring Editor: Ruby Richardson
Production Manager: Berta Steiner
Cover and text design by: Caliber Design Planning, Inc.

Typeset by: Bi-Comp, Inc.
Manufactured in the United States of America by: Halliday Lithograph

Library of Congress Cataloging in Publication Data

Morton, Richard F., 1924–
  A study guide to epidemiology and biostatistics.

  Includes bibliographical references and index.
  1. Epidemiology. 2. Medical statistics. I. Hebel,
J. Richard (John Richard), 1935–   II. Title.
RA651.M64   1984   614.4   83-23286
ISBN 0-8391-1974-7

Contents

Preface   *vii*
Acknowledgments   *ix*
How to Use This Book   *xi*
Goals and Objectives   *xiii*

1   **Investigation of an Epidemic**   **1**

2   **Measures of Mortality**   **19**

3   **Incidence and Prevalence**   **27**

4   **Measures of Risk**   **33**

    Self-Assessment 1   **37**

5   **Biological Variability**   **43**

6   **Probability**   **53**

7   **Screening**   **59**

8   **Sampling**   **67**

9   **Statistical Significance**   **73**

10   **Correlation**   **81**

    Self-Assessment 2   **89**

11   **Retrospective Studies**   **95**

12 **Prospective Studies** **103**

13 **Randomized Clinical Trials** **111**

14 **Association and Causation** **117**

Self-Assessment 3 **125**

Self-Assessment Final **131**

Answers to Self-Assessments **141**

Index *142*

Preface

The two disciplines, epidemiology and biostatistics, are receiving increasing recognition for their ubiquity in problem solving. This book provides coordinated instruction in these subjects.

The book is intended for students of the entire spectrum of the health sciences, including medicine, nursing, dentistry, pharmacy, public and community health, and allied health sciences. The scope and level are appropriate for professional schools, universities, four-year colleges, community colleges, and, in fact, any setting where courses in health sciences are taught. Our text is based upon a course given to second-year students at the University of Maryland School of Medicine. Our students have found this book an effective study guide. It has been used successfully for individual, self-paced instruction by selected students.

Our book has a distinct method, based upon pedagogic principles. The thirty objectives, expressed in behavioral terms, cite the concepts to be learned and the level at which students are expected to perform. There are three elements to the book, the first being the study notes. These may be read as the sole source of input to cover the material or they may be used to supplement attendance at a lecture series. These notes are not designed to replace or compete with existing textbooks of epidemiology and biostatistics, which are specifically referenced following each chapter. (The student is encouraged to augment his learning by reference to these books.) The second element is the exercises that accompany each chapter. The exercises encourage the student to immediately use his new-found knowledge, and this practice improves retention. Detailed feedback is provided in the exercise answers, which are amplified at points where we have learned that some students have difficulty. The third element in the instruction process is the multiple-choice examinations, which have the same scope and are on the same level that the student may expect to encounter in professional examinations. The student is challenged both progressively as the material is covered and comprehensively in a final examination.

vii

This new edition contains current data and covers three additional topics. Predictive value of a positive test has been included in the chapter on "Screening," and sample size considerations in the chapter on "Statistical Significance." The influence of informed consent is discussed in the chapter on "Randomized Clinical Trials."

Richard F. Morton
J. Richard Hebel

Acknowledgments

We would like to thank the students of the University of Maryland School of Medicine for providing us with the experience necessary to make this book possible.

How to Use This Book

To the student:

We suggest that, as you begin each chapter, you first read the accompanying study notes. If they are not sufficiently detailed, please read the standard textbooks listed in the Recommended Readings for that chapter, which are cited in ascending order of difficulty.

Following each chapter are exercises; you should answer the questions, preferably writing down your responses, before consulting the solutions provided. When the first third of the book is completed, you will encounter a multiple-choice self-assessment exam consisting of 20 questions. Complete the exam and score your efforts (answers are given on p. 141). You should score at least 60% before proceeding to the next chapters. If you should fail to achieve this level at your first attempt, we suggest that you restudy the sections with which you had difficulty. Similar self-assessment exams are provided following Chapters 10 and 14. A passing grade of 60% is also suggested for these. The final examination, covering all the objectives, may then be attempted. We suggest that 75% constitutes a passing grade on the total 100 questions, and that 90% indicates an honor grade.

To the instructor:

This book is versatile. It may be used as a course textbook for a formal lecture series given to large groups. It also has a role in a seminar series, freeing the instructor from didactic teaching, thereby enabling more complete discussion of relevant examples. It may be used as a vehicle for an independent study program wherein the faculty assumes the role of a tutor. The exclusive feature of our large question bank provides the instructor with a ready-made assessment instrument to monitor the progress of the students. Specific weaknesses may be identified and focal remediation given.

Goals and Objectives

Goals

After completing this study guide, the student will be able to:

1. Apply epidemiologic methods to evaluate the distribution and determinants of disease in the population.
2. Assess data by using biostatistical principles and evaluate conclusions based on such data.

Objectives

1. Interpret the distribution of disease in a population according to time, place, and person.
2. Describe the composition of a rate, in terms of the numerator and denominator, explain the relationship between them, and explain the use of rates for comparative purposes.
3. Define and compute an attack rate, and employ it to identify a vehicle of transmission in a common-source outbreak of disease.
4. Define:
   a. crude mortality rate
   b. specific mortality rate (age, sex, race, and cause)
   c. case fatality rate
   d. proportionate mortality ratio
   Cite one example of the correct use of each rate listed above, and interpret statements containing them.
5. State the reasons for adjustment of rates and interpret statements containing adjusted rates.
6. Define incidence and prevalence; state the relationship between them. Name the factors that may cause variation in each measurement. Give the uses of each rate.

7. Define absolute risk, relative risk, and attributable risk. Interpret statements that employ these terms.
8. State the purpose of a frequency distribution and cumulative frequency distribution in describing a set of biological measurements.
9. Define mean, median, mode, and percentile, and describe the features of a distribution that each characterizes.
10. Contrast the features of a normal (Gaussian) distribution with those of a skewed distribution.
11. Explain why the mean ±2 standard deviations is often used to establish the "normal range" and what practical difficulties might be encountered using this procedure in clinical practice.
12. Determine probabilities by using frequency distribution.
13. Explain what is meant by conditional probability.
14. Calculate the probability of complex events by applying the addition and multiplication rules.
15. Define sensitivity, specificity, and predictive value of a screening test and compute these measures given the necessary data.
16. Describe the selection of screening test criteria with respect to the natural history of the disease in question.
17. Use the standard error to compute 95% confidence limits for a mean or a proportion and interpret statements containing confidence limits.
18. Explain sampling bias and describe how random sampling operates to avoid bias in the process of data collection.
19. Distinguish between the standard deviation and the standard error and give one example of the use of each.
20. Interpret statements of statistical significance with regard to comparisons of means and frequencies and explain what is meant by a statement such as "$P < 0.05$."
21. Distinguish between the statistical significance of a result and its importance in clinical application.
22. Interpret the relationship between two variables as displayed on a scattergram, distinguishing between positive, negative, and zero correlation.
23. Explain the information provided by a regression equation as well as that provided by a correlation coefficient.
24. Interpret statements of statistical significance with regard to the correlation coefficient.
25. Distinguish between experimental and observational studies.
26. Describe the following types of epidemiologic studies:
    a. case-control
    b. prospective
    c. cross-sectional
    d. randomized clinical trials
27. Define cohort, and recognize a cohort effect when interpreting cross-sectional data.

28. Illustrate with one example the concept of multifactorial causation of disease.
29. Define the following types of association:
    a. artifactual
    b. noncausal
    c. causal
30. Distinguish between association and causation and list five criteria that support a causal inference.

1

Investigation of an Epidemic

Objectives Covered

1. Interpret the distribution of disease in a population according to time, place, and person.
2. Describe the composition of a rate, in terms of the numerator and denominator, explain the relationship between them, and explain the use of rates for comparative purposes.
3. Define and compute an attack rate, and employ it to identify a vehicle of transmission in a common-source outbreak of disease.

Study Notes

Epidemiology is the study of the distribution and determinants of disease. We try to find out who gets the disease and why. For example, is the disease more frequent among men or women, young or old, rich or poor, blacks or whites? Did they get the disease because of a genetic trait, an occupational exposure, or a lifestyle habit, such as cigarette smoking?

Epidemiology differs from clinical medicine in two important regards: First, epidemiologists study groups of people, not individuals. Second, epidemiologists study well people, in addition to sick people, and try to find out the crucial difference between those stricken and those spared. What is the trait common to the sick, yet rare in the well? Epidemiology weighs and balances, contrasts and compares. To determine if a study is an epidemiologic study look for a control or comparison group. To make a comparison, you need to develop a rate. A rate is computed as:

$$\frac{\text{events}}{\text{population at risk}}$$

It is usually expressed as events per 1,000 individuals, or some other convenient base.

The numerator is merely the number of people to whom something happened (i.e., they got sick or died) in the population at risk. The numerator must be derived (i.e., be a subset) of the denominator. The denominator (the population at risk) has to be all the people at risk for the event. For mortality, the denominator is the entire population, because death is a universal risk, but in pregnancy rates, for example, only females in the reproductive age group would comprise the denominator.

Attack Rate

An attack rate measures the proportion of the population that develops disease among the total exposed to a specific risk:

$$\text{attack rate} = \frac{\text{number of persons ill}}{\text{number of persons at risk}}$$

In an outbreak of food poisoning, attack rates are computed for all items ingested. These attack rates are computed for those people who are exposed (i.e., ate the item studied) and, most importantly, those who are not exposed (i.e., did not eat the item studied), as is illustrated by Table 1.

By inspecting attack rates for those who ate specific items, it is impossible to incriminate a single vehicle. Comparing the attack rates between those who ate and did not eat a specified food, however, is more

TABLE 1.   Differential Attack Rates of Illness According to Food Histories in an Epidemic of Food Poisoning

Food	Persons Who Ate Specified Food			Persons Who Did Not Eat Specified Food			Difference in Attack Rates
	Number	Number Ill	Attack Rate (%)	Number	Number Ill	Attack Rate (%)	
Turkey	133	97	73	25	2	8	+65
Dressing	121	88	73	37	11	30	+43
Potatoes and gravy	127	92	72	31	7	22	+50
Peas	105	77	73	53	22	41	+32
Rolls	66	50	76	92	49	53	+23
Margarine	66	50	76	92	49	53	+23
Salads	4	1	25	154	98	64	−39
Desserts	36	22	61	122	77	63	−2
Sandwich	11	1	9	147	98	67	−58
Coffee	98	59	60	60	40	67	−7
Milk	18	12	67	140	87	62	+5

Modified from Tong et al., 1962.

TABLE 2. Attack Rates for Food Combinations

	Ate Turkey			Did Not Eat Turkey		
	Number	Number Ill	Attack Rate (%)	Number	Number Ill	Attack Rate (%)
Ate potatoes and gravy	127	92	72	0	0	—
Did not eat potatoes and gravy	6	5	83	25	2	8

Modified from Tong et al., 1962.

informative. The last column on the right shows this difference. To distinguish between turkey, and potatoes and gravy, both of which show large differences in attack rates, it is necessary to cross-classify, as is shown in Table 2. A study of this table clearly incriminates turkey as the suspected vehicle.

Investigation of an Epidemic

An epidemic occurs when there are significantly more cases of the same disease than past experience would have predicted for that place, at that time, among that population. Disease in the individual may be considered the outcome of the interaction of three factors: agent, host, and environment. A triad, time, place, and person, is also used in the investigation of disease in the community.

Cases of the disease may be classified according to these three categories:

1. time, which includes date of onset
2. place, which includes dwelling and work place
3. personal characteristics, which include age, sex, and occupation

Scrutiny of the results of such classification enables one to recognize characteristics common among the sick and rare among the well.

Epidemic Curve

An epidemic curve gives a convenient pictorial depiction of the epidemic and certain limited deductions may be drawn. In a common-source outbreak, such as that just discussed, the time between the common exposure (e.g., the meal) and the peak of the cases approximates the incubation period of the disease. There are few or no secondary cases, and the curve is unimodal (see Figure 1).

However, in a typical infectious disease, such as measles, which is spread from person to person, the picture of propagation, as shown by an epidemic curve, is not so clear. In a closed community, such as a

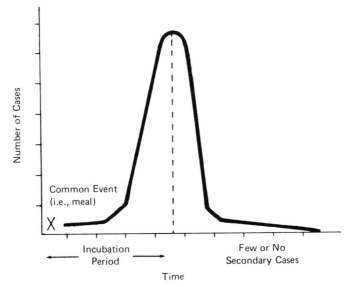

FIGURE 1   Common-Source Outbreak.

school, barracks, or ship, it may be possible to trace successive waves of propagation, each resulting in a new crop of cases, separated from the previous peak by an incubation period. The epidemic ceases when the supply of susceptibles is exhausted.

Analysis

When the data have been collected, they may be analyzed as follows:

a. Plot an epidemic curve. Incubation periods may be estimated if times of exposure are known.
b. Calculate attack rates for different age, sex, and occupation categories.
c. Plot the geographic distribution of cases by residence and/or work place.

On the basis of the analysis under a, b, and c above, a suspected vehicle may be identified. Attack rates may then be computed for those exposed and not exposed to this vehicle. However, sometimes this is not possible. For instance, in the investigation of a busy restaurant, the total exposed to a particular food is often unknown. In such instances, we compare, between the sick and a sample of the well, the proportions exposed to the suspected vehicle, as illustrated below.

At a restaurant food poisoning occurred in 30 people, among whom 24, or 80%, ate raw oysters. This proportion alone is insufficient to incriminate oysters. It is necessary to investigate a sample of those diners not afflicted. Suppose we find that in 30 well diners, only 3, or

10%, ate the oysters. This is convincing evidence to incriminate the oysters. Please note that the comparison above is between exposure rates among the sick and well, whereas in Table 1 the comparison is of attack rates between exposed and nonexposed.

Exercise: An Outbreak of Jaundice in a Rural Community[1]

Introduction

On Friday, May 17, 1968, a request to assist in the investigation of an outbreak of infectious hepatitis was extended to the Hepatitis Unit of the Center for Disease Control (CDC) in Atlanta, Georgia. It was learned that between April 30 and May 16, 1968, approximately 32 cases of infectious hepatitis had been reported to District #2 Health Department in North Trail, Michigan.

1. **Knowing that between April 30 and May 16, 1968, there were 32 cases of jaundice reported to the County Health Department, could one conclude that this is a problem of epidemic proportions? Why?**

Background

Lake County (Figure 2) is located in the northern portion of the lower peninsula of Michigan. The county has an area of 576 square miles and a population (1960 census) of 9,680—2,025 of whom live in North Trail, the county seat. The area is predominately rural, divided between farmland and forest.

The epidemic investigation was centered on the city of North Trail, in the southwestern portion of the county. There are only two other communities of notable size in Lake County—Spruce City, population 435, and Basco, population 308.

The remaining area is divided into 14 subdivisions, with the population being mostly in the low middle socioeconomic class; in the summer there is also a large tourist population.

Seven cases of infectious hepatitis were reported to the Michigan District #2 Health Department in the year prior to April 1968. Four of these cases occurred in one family outbreak in August 1967. The remaining three cases were scattered in time and no relationship could be established between them.

---

[1] The information in this section was drawn from an article in the *American Journal of Epidemiology* (Schoenbaum, S. C., Baker, O., and Jezek, Z. 1976. Vol. 104, No. 1, pp. 74–80). The place names have been changed.

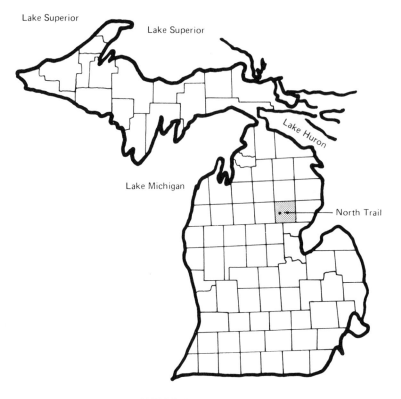

MICHIGAN

FIGURE 2   Location of Lake County, Michigan.

2. a. Are 32 cases in excess of normal expectancy?
   b. How does one establish whether this is greater than ex-
      pected?

Epidemic Investigation

By May 19, 39 cases of hepatitis had been reported. By May 25 the number had risen to 61, and by June 1 the last two cases were reported, bringing the total to 63.

The first step in the investigation consisted of personally interviewing all reported hepatitis victims. All interviews were conducted by the same two investigators at the patients' homes. Patients were questioned about the date of onset of illness, symptoms of illness, previous exposure to cases of hepatitis, visits out of the community, and history of receiving injections of blood products. In addition, information was obtained for all other members of the family concerning recent illnesses and the administration of gamma globulin. The patients and their families were

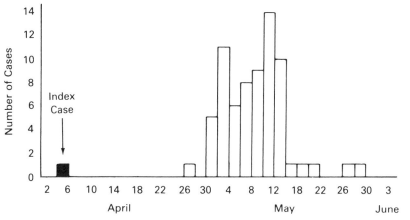

FIGURE 3   Cases of Infectious Hepatitis, April–May 1968, Lake County.

questioned about specific sources of water, milk, and food and attendance at large gatherings or public places. At the time of the interview, a
tap water sample was taken from each home for bacteriological analysis.

3. Ideally, what additional information should have been sought?

Epidemic Characteristics

Of Time

A total of 63 cases of infectious hepatitis were reported in Lake County
between April 1 and May 8, 1968 (Figure 3). Of these, 61 had date of
onset of illness between April 28 and May 26 (see Figure 3, which is an
epidemic curve).

**4. What inferences may be drawn regarding the probable time of
initial exposure to the infection?**

Of Person

Table 3 illustrates the age- and sex-specific attack rates of Lake County
cases with the date of onset of disease between April 28 and May 26.
Over all, the attack rate among males was almost twice as high as the
attack rate among females, 8.1 per 1,000 versus 4.5 per 1,000 population, respectively.

Forty-three (70%) of the total Lake County cases occurred in school
children, the remainder in the post-school children population. Thirty-
six of the 43 school children had attended the North Trail Public School.
New cases occurred each at St. Luke's School, the Spruce City School,
and the Basco School. There was one Lake County case at Brecken
School in neighboring Penton County.

TABLE 3.   Attack Rates by Age and Sex in Cases of Infectious Hepatitis—Lake County, April 28–May 26

Age Group	Total Population by Age	Number of Cases			Attack Rate Per 1,000 Population		
		Male	Female	Total	Male	Female	Total
0–4	1740	0	0	0	0.0	0.0	0.0
5–9	1000	2	2	4	3.7	4.5	4.0
10–14	989	12	6	18	22.2	13.4	18.2
15–19	868	16	7	23	35.9	16.6	26.5
20–24	494	1	3	4	4.2	11.8	8.1
25–29	455	0	1	1	0.0	4.6	2.2
30–34	435	3	0	3	14.1	0.0	6.9
35–39	545	1	2	3	4.0	6.7	5.5
40–44	540	2	0	2	7.4	0.0	3.7
45–49	588	1	0	1	3.4	0.0	1.7
50–54	526	2	0	2	7.6	0.0	3.8
55+	1500	0	0	0	0.0	0.0	0.0
Totals	9680	40	21	61	8.1	4.5	6.3

5. a. **How many victims were under 5 years old?**
    b. **Which decade of life had the highest attack rate?**
    c. **What hypothesis relative to time and person can one make at this point in this investigation?**

Of Place

Lake County has four school districts, two of which are extensions from adjacent Penton County. The largest district is the one served by the North Trail Public School (a single building complex located near downtown North Trail, serving 1,525 pupils in kindergarten through twelfth grade). Seventy percent of the pupils of this school use the school buses. North Trail also has a Roman Catholic parochial school with 240 pupils, grades 1 through 8. This school utilizes the same buses as the North Trail Public School. Table 4 shows attack rates by grade for North Trail Public School and St. Luke's School. The attack rates are uniformly low through grade 6, but beginning in grade 7 there is an increase in the attack rates in the public school. The peak attack rate, 8.6%, occurred in grade 10, followed by substantially lower attack rates in grades 11 and 12. There is a marked difference in the attack rates between the 7th and 8th grade classes of the public and parochial school.

6. **What can one conclude now with this information about the distribution of disease in terms of place?**

TABLE 4. Attack Rates by Grade and School in Cases of Infectious Hepatitis—Lake County, April 28–May 26

	North Trail Public School				Saint Luke's School		
Grade	Number in Class	Number Ill	Attack Rate (%)	Grade	Number in Class	Number Ill	Attack Rate (%)
Kind.	126	2	1.6				
1	128	0	0.0	1	37	1	2.7
2	121	0	0.0	2	41	1	2.4
3	107	0	0.0	3	37	0	0.0
4	106	2	1.9	4	26	0	0.0
5	120	1	0.8	5	30	0	0.0
6	111	1	0.9	6	32	0	0.0
7	110	3	2.7	7	26	0	0.0
8	120	6	5.0	8	21	0	0.0
9	143	7	4.9				
10	128	11	8.6				
11	112	1	0.9				
12	93	2	2.2				

Analysis Related to Age

Note that Table 3 gives the frequency distribution of hepatitis cases by age and that Table 4 gives it by school and grade.

7. **Why is it important to calculate attack rates by age? Note once again that the majority of cases in Table 3 fall within the age group between 10 and 19 years, which is confirmed by the attack rates.**

8. **Utilizing the information calculated about place and person, what conclusions can one draw now?**

Source of the Epidemic

Using the information concerning time, place, and person, the investigators gathered relevant information concerning the school population. Children who attend kindergarten through grade 6 are not allowed to leave the campus for lunch. They may eat food prepared at the school cafeteria or may bring a lunch from home. Children in Grades 7 through 12 at the North Trail High School, however, may leave the school during lunch hour. Since the school is only one block from the main street of North Trail, many students go downtown for lunch each day. St. Luke's School, however, does not allow any of its students, grades 1 through 8, to leave the campus for lunch. All parochial school students must eat in the school cafeteria or bring lunch from home.

TABLE 5.   Exposure History of 41 Hepatitis Victims, Ages 10–19, Lake County, May, 1968

Food or Water	Yes	No	Unknown	Percent Known Exposed
Restaurant A	15	25	1	36.6
Restaurant B	17	23	1	41.5
North Trail Dairy Queen	28	12	1	68.3
Spruce City Dairy Queen	8	32	1	19.5
North Trail Bakery	37	3	1	90.2
North Trail municipal water supply	36	5	0	87.8

Convinced that there was a common source of exposure, the investigators began to look for a vehicle of transmission. The first major sources investigated were those of food and water. Table 5 gives an exposure history of 41 hepatitis victims, ages 10 to 19, in Lake County in May 1968.

9. a. From the information given in Table 5, what hypothesis can be formed about the source of the infection?
    b. Is this type of data alone sufficient to identify a single source?

Food History of Well Individuals

Up until this point, the investigator concentrated upon the sick individuals in the population. The attack rates were computed for specific food sources. To build a case, it is now necessary to examine food sources in the well population. By comparing the differential rates of exposure to sources between the well and the ill populations, one should be able to further elucidate the true source of the infection.

10. a. Examine Table 6. When the six listed exposures are compared, which source shows the largest differential between well and ill?
     b. Explain the high exposure rates to water in both the sick and well groups.

Milk Source

All commercial milk sold in Lake County comes from dairies located outside the county. None of the commercially produced milk in Michigan is limited to Lake County alone.

11. What conclusions can one draw about milk possibly being the source of the contamination?

TABLE 6. Comparison of the Exposure History of 41 Victims of Hepatitis A in the 10–19-Year-Old Age Group with the Exposure History of a Group of 56 Well Household Members in the 10–19-Year-Old Age Group, Lake County, May 1968

	Hepatitis Victims			
	Number Yes	Number No	Number Unknown	Percent Known Exposure
Restaurant A	15	25	1	36.6
Restaurant B	17	23	1	41.5
North Trail Dairy Queen	28	12	1	68.3
Spruce City Dairy Queen	8	32	1	19.5
North Trail Bakery	37	3	1	90.2
North Trail water	30	5	0	87.8
	Well household members			
Restaurant A	22	31	3	39.3
Restaurant B	15	39	2	26.8
North Trail Dairy Queen	39	17	0	69.6
Spruce City Dairy Queen	6	50	0	10.7
North Trail Bakery	26	29	1	46.4
North Trail water	51	4	1	91.1

Food Sources

Common exposure to a food item could explain the characteristics of this common-source outbreak. The only food items prepared and consumed locally are the foods served in the restaurants, salads sold in the delicatessens, Dairy Queen ice cream, and baked goods. Most of these products have been eaten at some time by the majority of the local residents. Almost all the cases who lived in Lake County gave a history of eating baked goods from the North Trail Bakery. However, it was impossible, from this information alone, to determine whether the bakery was the source of the epidemic or simply a very popular establishment in town.

12. Study Figure 4. How do these data aid in the investigation?

Review of Case Histories

To further study the problem, the investigators sought victims who lived outside Lake County. In any such investigation, detailed case histories often revealed supporting evidence.

Case 1 The reported victim was a 45-year-old female school teacher who lives in Purley, a town on Lake Huron, 60 miles from North Trail. Her only contacts with Lake County were when she passed through North Trail on March 20, April 5, and April 14 on the way to

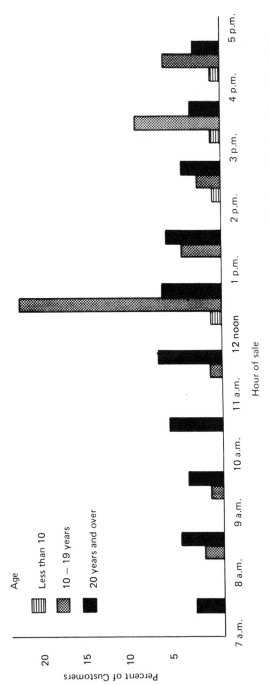

FIGURE 4 Percent of Total Persons Patronizing North Trail Bakery by Hour of Sale and by Age, June 3, 1968.

visit her father who lived on Lake Michigan's shore of the state. She stopped only on the first two occasions. On March 20, she had only a cup of coffee in a North Trail restaurant. On April 5, she bought some cupcakes and a coffee cake. On May 5, she became ill with hepatitis.

Case 2   A 35-year-old housewife who lives in Detroit, Michigan.

Case 3   The 8-year-old daughter of the patient in Case 2.

Case 4   A 49-year-old housewife who lives in Potomac. She is the sister-in-law of Case 2 and the aunt of Case 3. Both Case 2's family and Case 4's family own summer cottages in Lake County (10 to 15 miles from North Trail). They went to their cottages on April 8, 9, and 10 to open them for the season. At no time did Case 4 or Case 3 go in or near the city of North Trail. On April 9, Case 4 took care of Case 2's children while Case 2 went into the city to conduct some business. At that time Case 2 bought some pastries at the North Trail Bakery to bring to the cottage for lunch. All three cases ate the same kind of glazed donut. Case 2 and Case 3 became ill on May 7th and Case 4 became ill on May 11. No other member of either family had the same kind of pastry and no other member of either family is known to have been ill since being in Lake County.

Case 5   Case 5 is a 35-year-old mother of six who purchased assorted glazed and iced products at the North Trail Bakery on April 6. She took the baked products home, where she and her two older daughters, Cases 6 and 7, ate some of them. Her two sons, Cases 8 and 9, returned home later in the day and consumed all but one glazed item. Still later, Case 10 and her 5-year-old twin came home and, after a dispute, Case 10 won possession of the glazed delicacy. She became ill, but her twin did not. The father, who was away at work throughout the day, did not eat any of the bakery goods and remained well.

13. Are the above data compatible with the bakery being the source of infection?

The occurrence of infectious hepatitis one month after direct exposure to the North Trail Bakery was illustrated by Case 1. Cases 3 and 4 showed that only contact with baked products could be associated with infectious hepatitis, because they had no contact with the North Trail municipal water supply, with any of the restaurants in North Trail, or with any other local food-handling establishment. None of these four cases had any history of contact with persons known to have infectious hepatitis or jaundice. None had a history of infections or administration of blood products within six months prior to the onset of illness and none had a history of recent ingestion of shellfish.

14. What would your next step in the investigation be?

One of the cases in Lake County was a baker's assistant. This 34-year-old white male is reported physically and mentally handicapped. He visited his physician on April 6, 1968, complaining of "vomiting and a cold." His wife visited the same physician two days later complaining of nausea and generalized headaches. The patient continued to work until April 11, when the diagnosis of infectious hepatitis was made. Co-workers at the bakery reported that the patient had dark urine for at least four days before he stopped working. He did not return to work until April 23. Figure 3 shows the complete epidemic. Note that the baker's assistant is the initial case (in black).

15. a. Does the epidemic curve reveal the incubation period for hepatitis?
   b. Does this curve still support a common source of infection?
16. Knowing that infectious hepatitis virus is killed by heat, what further investigation would one undertake to confirm the source of the virus?

Investigation of the Bakery

The North Trail Bakery has served the region for 34 years. It makes a variety of breads, pastries, donuts, cookies, pies, and cakes. Besides over-the-counter sales in downtown North Trail, the bakery supplies all sweet rolls and donuts and some of the bread to each of the restaurants in the North Trail area and to grocery stores in Lake County.

The baker's assistant helps in practically every process of the baked goods. In particular, he is responsible for making and glazing donuts and for icing much of the pastry. Observation by investigators revealed that icing was spread on the pastries by hand and items to be glazed were dipped into the glaze by hand. Since the pastry is not cooked further after glazing or icing, these processes are likely points of contamination.

Both glaze and icing may be kept for several days and old batches may be used to start new ones. Bakery products not sold in one day may be sold in the next business day as "day-old pastries" or may be frozen for sale in the next one to two weeks. Therefore, contaminated foods could be available for consumption over a period of several days or weeks. In the midst of the epidemic investigation, as it became clear that the bakery was an increasingly likely source, a blood sample was taken from each person who worked in the bakery to ascertain whether or not there were any cases of hepatitis present at the time in the bakery employees.

An SGPT (an enzyme test for liver function) was performed on each blood sample and in all instances the SGPT was within normal limits. Because the epidemic curve showed that the outbreak was ending at this time (June 3) and because there was no elevated SGPT found, the bakery was permitted to remain open.

17. **Do you agree with this decision? Support your view.**
18. **Since none of the bakery employees appeared ill, why were SGPT performed?**

Control Measures

Serum gamma globulin was immediately offered to all residents, and 7,000 to 8,000 doses were distributed after June 3, 1968.

19. a. **Since the epidemic had ended, why was it necessary to administer the gamma globulin?**
    b. **How would you evaluate the effectiveness of this control measure?**

Exercise Answers

1. **One cannot determine whether or not 32 cases of jaundice constitute an epidemic unless one knows how many cases to expect in that place during that time.**

2. a. **Yes.**
   b. **To be sure these cases are in excess of what may be expected, one could apply a statistical test. However, usually the fact that four times the annual number of cases had occurred in a very short space of time is sufficient to warrant an investigation.**

3. **The additional information needed is similar data on a group of well individuals.**

4. **We may assume that these cases were all exposed on or about the first week of April, about 30 days before peak.**

5. a. **No cases under 5 years old.**
   b. **10–19 year olds had the highest attack rates.**
   c. **The attack rate is highest in males. The cases occur during a limited time period. The epidemic appears to be due to a common source to which children under school age were not exposed.**

6. **All but 8 of the cases occurred in the North Trail school district. This suggests that the common experience of most cases may relate to attendance in North Trail schools.**

7. Age as well as place may give clues to the mechanism of spread and the common experience that caused the outbreak. Age is also indicative of immune status from previous exposures.

8. The epidemic occurred primarily in North Trail School in the junior and senior high school children.

9. a. No inference can be drawn from Table 5, since there is neither a comparison group without disease nor their exposure history. We suspect that it would be one of the sources with high attack rates, e.g., Dairy Queen, bakery, or water. Maybe all people, sick or well, use the water and bakery, so that is why these percentages are high. Investigate these three further.
   b. No.

10. a. The investigator used well household members as controls and found no difference in water sources and exposure to Dairy Queen, but a big difference between the exposure of victims and the exposure of controls to the North Trial Bakery.
    b. Water history was high in both groups since all persons in the same household usually have similar water supply, except possibly in rural areas where wells are used.

11. Milk supply is not the problem because 1) there are no cases among young children, who also receive milk, and 2) there is no epidemic in the other counties where the same milk is sold.

12. Figure 4 indicates that at lunchtime and again after school, a very high percentage of the customers of the bakery are 10 to 19 years old.

13. Yes—all these cases outside the county can be traced to a known exposure to bakery products. As noted in the discussion, two cases were exposed to nothing else from North Trail.

14. The next step is to try to determine the source in the bakery.

15. a. From the curve one can infer that the incubation period is 24 to 28 days.
    b. Yes.

16. Ascertain if the initial case handled bakery products that had uncooked material. Did the victims consume uncooked bakery material?

17. As usually happens by the time of the investigation, the epidemic is over; there were no signs of active disease in current workers. However, the bakery should be warned about the glaz-

ing procedures in order to minimize the chance of subsequent problems.

18. SGPT elevation could indicate liver dysfunction, which might indicate a subclinical case of hepatitis.

19. a. Gamma globulin was administered to prevent any secondary spread of hepatitis. There were very few cases after mid-May, so use of globulin early in June might have been a little late. However, the epidemic could have been protracted at a low level for several more months through family contacts.

    b. Compare exposed individuals who have and have not received globulin in order to determine the number of cases of hepatitis, clinical and subclinical.

Recommended Readings

1. Mausner, J. S., and Bahn, A. K. 1984. *Epidemiology—An Introductory Text,* second edition, chapters 6 and 12. W. B. Saunders Company, Philadelphia.
2. Lilienfeld, A. M., and Lilienfeld, D. E. 1980. *Epidemiology: Foundations,* second edition, chapter 7. Oxford University Press, New York.

Reference

Tong, J. L., Engle, M., Cullingford, J. S., Shimp, D. T., and Love, C. E. 1962. Am. J. Pub. Health. 52:976.

2

Measures
of Mortality

Objectives Covered

4. Define:
   a. crude mortality rate
   b. specific mortality rate (age, sex, race, and cause)
   c. case fatality rate
   d. proportionate mortality ratio
   Cite one example of the correct use of each rate listed above, and interpret statements containing them.
5. State the reasons for adjustment of rates and interpret statements containing adjusted rates.

Study Notes

Crude death rate =

$$\frac{\text{all deaths during a calendar year}}{\text{population at midyear}} \times 1,000 = \text{deaths per 1,000}$$

This crude rate expresses the actual observed death rate in a population under study and it should always be the starting point for further development of adjusted rates.

The crude death rate measures the proportion of the population dying every year or the number of deaths in the community per 1,000 population (by convention usually taken as the population at midyear). It is important to recognize that the crude death rate reflects the effect of two factors:

1. the probability of dying (this factor is correctly measured by the age-specific mortality rates explained below)
2. the age characteristics or age distribution of the population under consideration.

Because the crude death rate is a composite figure reflecting two factors, namely, specific mortality rates and population composition, it is necessary to disentangle the two factors before meaningful comparisons can be made between population groups.

Mortality and Age

Age is the most important characteristic governing the distribution of disease. Before disease experience in two populations can be compared, account must be taken of differences in age composition. Crude death rates were 10.9 per 1,000 population in Florida in 1981 and 4.4 per 1,000 in Alaska in the same year. The 148% higher death rate in Florida is due to its older population, compared with the younger population of Alaska.

Age-Specific Death Rates

Because of the profound effect of age on mortality, it is necessary to construct death rates for each age group and to use these rates for comparison. Table 7 shows the crude death rate and the age-specific death rate in Baltimore City. A paradox is seen. The whites in Baltimore have a higher overall death rate than the blacks—15.2 and 9.8, respectively. On the other hand, blacks suffer higher age-specific death rates in every age group. What is the explanation for this seeming contradiction? Age distribution is the answer. The population of Baltimore City consists of old whites and young blacks.

Age-Adjusted Death Rates

When there are differences in age distribution for the groups we wish to compare, age-adjusted rates should be used. To understand what is meant by an age-adjusted death rate, it must first be recognized that a crude death rate may be expressed as a weighted sum of age-specific death rates. Each component of the sum has the following form:

proportion of the population in the age group × age-specific death rate

TABLE 7. Death Rates per 1,000 Population by Age and Race in Baltimore City, 1972

	All Ages	Under 1 Year	1–4	5–17	18–44	45–65	65 and Over
White	15.2	13.5	0.6	0.4	1.5	10.7	59.7
Black	9.8	22.6	1.0	0.5	3.6	18.8	61.1

Source: Baltimore City Statistics.

TABLE 8. Age-Specific Death Rates per 1,000

Community	Young	Old
A	4	16
B	5	20

The crude death rate is age-adjusted by replacing the first term in each of the products by the corresponding age proportion for a standard population (often the U.S. population for a recent year is taken as the standard). This procedure is best illustrated by the following example.

Community A has a population composed of one-half young people and one-half old people. Community B has two-thirds young people and one-third old people in its population. The age-specific death rates in the communities are shown in Table 8.

From this information we can determine the crude death rates, as follows:

crude death rate in A = (1/2)(4) + (1/2)(16) = 10 per 1,000

crude death rate in B = (2/3)(5) + (1/3)(20) = 10 per 1,000

Notice that although the probability of dying is lower for A in both age groups, the crude death rates are the same. This is because A has an older population than B.

Now we shall adjust the death rates for age using a standard population composition of one-third young and two-thirds old, arbitrarily chosen:

age-adjusted death rate for A = (1/3)(4) + (2/3)(16) = 12 per 1,000

age-adjusted death rate for B = (1/3)(5) + (2/3)(20) = 15 per 1,000

The age-adjusted rates reflect only the probability of dying for these communities and thus we have a comparison that is not influenced by the age composition of the populations.

In summary, rates are adjusted in order to remove the effect of a factor for which the adjustment is being made. However, it is always necessary first of all to look at the overall crude rates because they represent events. An adjusted rate gives an accurate comparison but does not reveal the underlying raw data, which are shown by the crude rate.

Race- and Sex-Specific Death Rates

Males have a higher mortality rate than females. In 1980, the age-adjusted death rate per 1,000 for males in the U.S. was 7.8, whereas for females it was only about half that, namely 4.3. Now, because these rates are age-adjusted, they cannot be explained by age differences and they must relate to sex differences. The male excess holds in both whites and blacks. In whites the rate is 7.5 for males versus 4.1 for females, whereas in blacks it is 11.1 for males versus 6.3 for females. The explanation for the higher overall mortality rate in males lies in the higher rates they suffer in the leading causes of death: cardiovascular and respiratory diseases, cancer, and accidents.

Cause-Specific Death Rates

Death rates for any specific disease, such as heart disease, may be stated for the entire population or for any age, race, or sex subgroup. Cause-specific death rates are computed as:

$$\frac{\text{deaths assigned to the specified disease during a calendar year}}{\text{population at midyear}} \times 100{,}000$$

[handwritten annotations: "or", "100,000" crossed out, "1 000" and "100,000" written]

and so are expressed as deaths per 100,000 population per year, e.g., for diseases of the heart 336 per 100,000 population in the USA in 1980. Diseases of the heart are typical of many diseases in that the death rate shows a differential between the sexes. In order to express these differences more clearly, age-adjusted rates by sex are used so that cause-specific death rates are shown as:

> Diseases of the heart—age-adjusted mortality rates by sex for the USA in 1980, per 100,000 population
>
> Males—280
> Females—140

Case Fatality Rate

$$\frac{\text{The number of deaths due to the disease in a specified period of time}}{\text{The number of cases of the disease in the same period in time}} \times 100$$

This measure represents the probability of death among diagnosed cases, or the killing power of a disease. It is typically used in acute infectious disease such as Acquired Immune Deficiency Syndrome (AIDS). Its usefulness for chronic diseases (even when, as with tuberculosis, they are infectious) is limited, because the period from onset to death is typically long and variable. The case fatality rate for the same disease may vary in different epidemics as the balance between agent, host, and environment alters.

Proportionate Mortality Ratio (PMR)

This measure is used to demonstrate the proportion of the overall mortality that may be ascribed to a specific cause. Thus, the definition of PMR is:

$$\frac{\text{the deaths assigned to the disease in a certain year}}{\text{the total deaths in the population in the same year}} \times 100$$

The use of this statistic is to display the percentage of deaths due to the cause under study, usually in a certain age and sex group compared with a different age group in the same sex group. For example, white males ages 20 to 24, who have a PMR due to motor vehicle accidents of 37% and a PMR due to arteriosclerotic heart disease of 2%, can be compared to white males ages 50 to 54, who have a PMR due to motor vehicle accidents of 2.4% and a PMR due to arteriosclerotic heart disease of 40%. The PMR is often used to emphasize the importance of the contribution of one cause-specific mortality to overall mortality. For example, in 1980 in the U.S. the proportionate mortality of heart disease was 38%. This means that 38% of all deaths, regardless of age, sex, or race, could be ascribed to diseases of the heart, making it, of course, the leading cause of death, with a proportionate mortality rate almost twice that of cancer, which is in second place at 21%. However, note that the statistic tells one nothing about the actual rate involved.

Exercise

1. There were 1,986,000 deaths in the U.S. in 1982. What additional information is required to compute the crude mortality rate?

2. The crude death rate has fluctuated moderately in New York City over the past 40 years, yet the age-adjusted rate has fallen by 42% (Table 9). What is the most probable explanation?

TABLE 9. Crude and Age-Adjusted Death Rates from All Causes per 1,000 Population, New York City and the United States, 1940–1980

Year	New York City		United States	
	Age-Adj.	Crude	Age-Adj.	Crude
1940	11.3	10.2	10.8	10.8
1950	8.9	10.0	8.4	9.6
1960	8.1	11.1	7.6	9.5
1970	7.7	11.2	7.1	9.5
1980	6.6	10.8	5.9	8.9

3. In 1970, the crude death rate (all causes) for Guyana (a developing country in South America) was 6.8 per 1,000, for the United States it was 9.4 per 1,000.
   a. Can the lower crude death rate in Guyana be explained by the fact that the United States has a larger population? Explain your answer.
   b. Give the most probable explanation for the lower crude death rate in Guyana.

4. Crude and age-adjusted death rates (per 100,000 persons) from "arteriosclerotic and degenerative heart diseases" are shown for Chile and the U.S. for 1967 (Table 10).

TABLE 10.

	Crude Rates	Age-Adjusted Rates
Chile	67.4	58.2
United States	316.3	131.4
Ratio, United States : Chile	4.7	2.3

Which of the two rates is preferable for comparing the death rate from heart disease in the two countries? Why? Why do the ratios of the crude and age-adjusted rates for the two countries differ?

5. A city contains 100,000 people (45,000 males and 55,000 females), and 1,000 people die per year (600 males and 400 females). There were 50 cases (40 males and 10 females) of lung cancer per year, of whom 45 died (36 males and 9 females). Compute:
   a. Crude mortality rate
   b. Sex-specific mortality rate
   c. Cause-specific mortality rate for lung cancer
   d. Case fatality rate for lung cancer
   e. PMR for lung cancer

Exercise Answers

1. The total U.S. midyear population in 1982, which was estimated to be 230,930,230.

   This gives a crude mortality rate of $\dfrac{1,986,000}{230,930,230}$

   $$\times\ 1,000 = 8.6 \text{ per } 1,100.$$

2. The crude death rate is not the best measure of trends in mortality since it assumes a stable age composition in the population. The age composition of New York City has changed over the past 40 years, with an increasing proportion of the population being in the older age groups. An age-adjusted rate should be used for comparison, which shows a steady fall. Similar patterns are found in U.S. mortality rates.

3. a. The fact that the population of the U.S. is larger than that of Guyana cannot explain a difference in rates, since the death rate refers to number of deaths per 1,000 population in both countries.

   b. Age-specific death rates are higher in Guyana, but the population in Guyana is younger. High age-specific death rates in the first decades of life, typical of developing countries, can lead to a relatively young population, because comparatively few people survive to live to an old age, thus giving a relative deficiency of old people. Thus, paradoxically, the crude death rate in developing countries is low, despite high age-specific death rates, because of the small proportion of elderly persons.

4. Age-adjusted rates are preferable. Crude death rates reflect not only age-specific death rates but also the age composition of the population. Since Chile, like Guyana, has a younger population than the United States, age-adjusted rates are needed for comparing the risk of death from heart disease in the two countries. When differences in age composition are removed by the adjustment, the death rate from heart disease in the United States is only 2.3 times that of Chile, rather than 4.7.

5. a. $1,000/100,000 \times 1000 = 10$ per 1,000.
   b. $600/45,000 \times 1000 = 13.3$ per 1,000 for males.
      $400/55,000 \times 1000 = 7.3$ per 1,000 for females.
   c. $45/100,000 \times 1000 = 0.45$ per 1,000.
   d. $45/50 \times 100 = 90\%$.
   e. $45/1,000 \times 100 = 4.5\%$.

Recommended Readings

1. Mausner, J. S., and Bahn, A. K. 1984. *Epidemiology—An Introductory Text*, second edition, chapters 3, 4, and 5. W. B. Saunders Company, Philadelphia.
2. Lilienfeld, A. M., and Lilienfeld, D. E. 1980. *Epidemiology: Foundations*, second edition, chapters 4, 5, and 6. Oxford University Press, New York.

3

Incidence
and Prevalence

Objective Covered

6. Define incidence and prevalence; state the relationship between them. Name the factors that may cause variation in each measurement. Give the uses of each rate.

Study Notes

Incidence and prevalence are the two major measurements of disease.

Incidence rates are designed to measure the rate at which people without a disease develop the disease during a specific period of time, i.e., the number of NEW cases of a disease in a population over a period of time. Prevalence rates measure the number of people in a population who have the disease at a given point in time. These rates are defined as follows:

$$\text{incidence rate} = \frac{\text{number of new cases of a disease over a period of time}}{\text{population at risk of developing the disease}}$$

$$\text{prevalence rate} = \frac{\text{total number of cases of a disease at a given time}}{\text{total population}}$$

The time referred to in the numerator of the prevalence rate may be a period of time such as a year or a specific time point such as January 1, 1984. In the former case, the term "period prevalence" is used, while in the latter it is "point prevalence."

Incidence measures the appearance of disease, prevalence measures the existence of disease.

Incidence means NEW.

Prevalence means ALL.

Incidence reflects only the rate of disease occurrence. A change in incidence means there is a change in the balance of etiological factors, either some naturally occurring fluctuation or possibly the application of an effective prevention program. Incidence is of importance to the researcher seeking etiology.

Prevalence, however, depends on two factors—the incidence and the duration of disease. Thus, a change in disease prevalence may reflect a change in incidence or outcome or both. For example, improvements in therapy, by preventing death but at the same time not producing recovery, may give rise to the apparently paradoxical effect of an increase in prevalence of the disease. Decrease in prevalence may result not only from a decrease in incidence, but also from a shortening of the duration of disease through either more rapid recovery or more rapid death. Further, if duration decreased sufficiently, a decrease in prevalence could take place despite an increase in incidence. Figure 5 illustrates that level of prevalence (all cases) is increased by incidence (new cases) and decreased by recovery and death.

Prevalence is the product of incidence times duration. This relationship is most apparent in a stable, chronic disease. In this case the incidence may be derived, provided the prevalence and duration are known.

Prevalence is used by health planners because it measures the need for treatment and hospital beds and aids in planning health facilities and manpower needs. Prevalence may be determined by a single survey; by

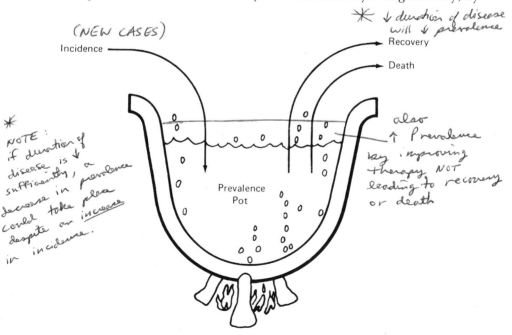

FIGURE 5 The Relationship between Incidence and Prevalence.

contrast, <u>incidence rates are difficult to measure</u>. A defined population,
initially free of the disease in question, must be followed forward for a
period of time in order to ascertain the rate of appearance of new cases.
Incidence rates are used to make statements about the probability or risk
of disease. Incidence rates of disease are compared among population
groups with different exposures or attributes in order to measure the
influence such factors may have on the occurrence of disease. Thus,
relative risk estimates are obtained (see Chapter 4).

Prospective

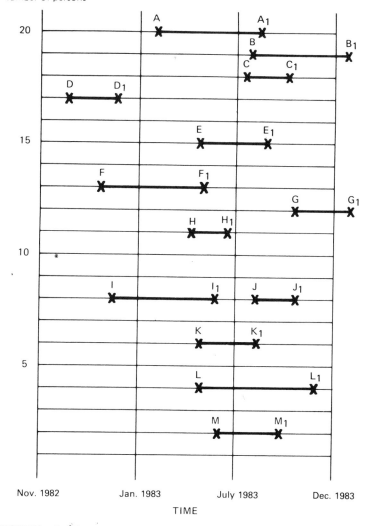

Number of persons

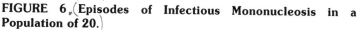

FIGURE 6. **(Episodes of Infectious Mononucleosis in a Population of 20.)**

Exercise

1. Each heavy black line between the X's on Figure 6 represents an episode of infectious mononucleosis, and each line represents a person (so that there is a defined population of 20). For 1983 compute, for mononucleosis:
   a. the incidence
   b. the period prevalence
   Assume a survey is conducted in July 1983; what point prevalence will result?

2. From the data in Table 11, compute the average duration, in years, of the five chronic neurological conditions listed.

$$P = I \times D \qquad D = \frac{P}{I}$$

TABLE 11. Prevalence and Incidence of Selected Neurological Diseases in Rochester, Minnesota

Disease	Rates per 100,000 Population	
	Prevalence	Incidence
Epilepsy	376	30.8
Multiple sclerosis	55	5.0
Parkinsons' disease	157	20.0
Motor neuron disease	7	1.7
CNS neoplasms	69	17.3

3. Assume that the prevalence of coronary heart disease decreases after age 70, while its incidence continues to increase with age. What is the most probable explanation for the divergence of these rates?

Exercise Answers

1. a. 10/20 or 50%. (The episode $J-J_1$ is counted as contributing to incidence in 1983, although it appears to be a reinfection.)
   b. 10 new + 1 old = prevalent cases/20 population. The period prevalence in 1983 = 11/20 = 55%.
   Point prevalence in July = 5 cases/20 population = 25%.

2. Epilepsy—12.2; multiple sclerosis—11; Parkinsons'—7.8; motor neuron disease—4.1; CNS neoplasm—4.0.

3. Patients over age 70 who develop coronary heart disease have shorter survival times than the younger patients.

Recommended Readings

1. Mausner, J. S., and Bahn, A. K. 1984. *Epidemiology—An Introductory Text,* second edition, chapters 3, 4, and 5. W. B. Saunders Company, Philadelphia.
2. Lilienfeld, A. M., and Lilienfeld, D. E. 1980. *Epidemiology: Foundations,* second edition, chapters 4, 5, and 6. Oxford University Press, New York.

4

Measures of Risk

Objective Covered

7. Define absolute risk, relative risk, and attributable risk. Interpret statements that employ these terms.

Study Notes

Relative and Attributable Risk

Relative and attributable risk are two measures of the association between exposure to a particular factor and risk of a certain outcome:

$$\text{relative risk} = \frac{\text{incidence rate among exposed}}{\text{incidence rate among nonexposed}}$$

Ratios not rates

$$\text{attributable risk} = \text{incidence rate among exposed} - \text{incidence rate among nonexposed}$$

This is sometimes expressed as a percentage of the incidence rate among the exposed, i.e.,

$$\frac{\text{incidence rate among exposed} - \text{incidence rate among nonexposed}}{\text{incidence rate among exposed}} \times 100$$

The absolute risk is synonymous with incidence and means the rate of occurrence of the condition or disease. It is the basic rate from which relative and attributable risk are derived. The clinician uses the relative risk, which expresses the risk of one group with a factor (males, hypertensives, cigarette smokers, etc.) compared to the risk of a reference group without such a factor (i.e., females, normotensives, nonsmokers). Relative risk is the ratio of the incidence of the group with the factor to the incidence of the group without the factor. Thus, it is not itself a rate but merely a ratio and does not indicate the incidence of disease, but it does tell the clinician how much the risk for his patient (the smoker) is increased (compared with a nonsmoker). Thus, his patient may be in a high risk group for a disease (by virtue of smoking), and a prescriptive screening test might be indicated to detect early asymptomatic disease. Also, the relative risk indicates the benefit that might accrue to the patient if the factor is removed, i.e., it measures the decrease in risk to be anticipated for the sacrifice involved in behavior change (stopping smoking). However, the relative risk does not measure the probability that someone with the factor will develop the disease. For example, if the relative risk associated with the presence of the factor is 10, this merely means that the probability for the disease is 10 times higher than in someone without the factor. The individual with the factor might still have a very remote chance of getting the disease, if the disease is rare. It has been shown that women who have used oral contraceptives for a long time have a high relative risk of developing liver cell adenoma. However, the underlying incidence of this disease is so small that the increased risk assumed by the users is insignificant in comparison to the benefits gained. It is especially important to bear this point in mind when the relative risk has been determined from a retrospective study (see Chapter 11). This is because this design does not yield incidence rates for either the exposed or the nonexposed groups. Thus, the relative risk estimate for those exposed is merely a multiple of an unknown incidence rate among those not exposed.

Relative risk also measures the strength of an association between a factor and a certain outcome; thus, a high relative risk points towards causation and is useful in research for the etiology of disease.

Attributable risk measures the amount of the absolute risk (incidence) that can be attributed to one particular factor (i.e., smoking). It is computed by taking the incidence rate of the group with the factor (smokers) and subtracting the rate for the group without the factor (nonsmokers). The excess suffered by the smokers is the attributable risk due to smoking. As defined above, the attributable risk indicates the excess of disease due to a factor in that subgroup of the population which is exposed to the factor. If we replace "incidence rate among exposed" in the formula for attributable risk with "incidence rate in the total population," we have the population attributable risk. The population attributable risk is generally of significance to public health authorities, as it measures the potential benefit to be expected if the exposure could be reduced in the population.

Clinical Implications

Although a factor may have a high relative risk, with reference to a common outcome or disease, if that factor is found only rarely in the population, the impact on the population will be small. For example, patients with familial multiple polyposis have a high relative risk for cancer of the large bowel, with a relative risk > 20 (i.e., they are more than 20 times as likely to develop large bowel cancer than those without familial polyposis), but the incidence of large bowel cancer due to familial multiple polyposis is very small because the attribute is rare. Therefore, it is necessary that a factor both have a high relative risk and be prevalent in the population in order for it to influence the incidence of the disease in the population.

Risk estimates are probability statements, and it must be remembered that 1) all those exposed to the factor do not develop the disease, they merely have an increased probability of doing so; and 2) some who have not been exposed to the factor will develop the disease.

Exercise

1. **From the data in Table 12, compute:**
   a. relative risk of smokers versus nonsmokers
   b. attributable risk for smokers

TABLE 12.

	Death Rates, from Lung Cancer, per 1,000 Persons Age 35 or More, per Year
Nonsmokers	0.07
Cigarette smokers	0.96

2. **Explain your answers to (a) and (b) above in narrative form.**

3. **What are the uses of relative risk**
   a. to the clinician?
   b. to the researcher?

4. **What are the uses of attributable risk**
   a. to the physician responsible for prevention programs?
   b. to the physician responsible for health planning for large groups?

5. **a. What does absolute risk measure?**
   b. When is it used?

6. **Males age 35 who are heavy cigarette smokers have a relative risk for lung cancer of 14. Compute the probability of a male cigarette smoker age 35 developing lung cancer per year.**

Exercise Answers

1. a. **0.96/0.07 = 13.7.**
   b. **0.96 − 0.07 = 0.89.**

2. a. **Cigarette smokers, over 35 years of age, are 13.7 times more likely to die from lung cancer than nonsmokers.**
   b. **Of the overall rate of deaths from lung cancer in cigarette smokers (0.96), 0.89 is attributable to cigarette smoking, or the percent attributable risk of lung cancer due to cigarette smoking is 0.89/0.96 × 100 = 93%.**

3. a. **Relative risk tells the clinician the size of the excess risk that his patient with exposure to a factor (i.e., hypertension, high serum cholesterol) runs, compared to a patient without exposure to such a factor. Relative risk enables the clinician to identify patients at high risk of certain outcomes. It does not provide the clinician with the absolute risk.**
   b. **The relative risk measures the strength of an association; thus a high relative risk suggests etiology or causality.**

4. a. **Attributable risk measures the impact that removal of a certain factor may have on the incidence of disease; therefore, prevention programs can be justified on the basis of a large attributable risk.**
   b. **Identification of attributable risks for various exposures in certain diseases aids in rational planning for health services.**

5. a. **It measures incidence, or rate of occurrence.**
   b. **It is used in actuarial or predictive situations.**

6. **Given the relative risk alone, it is impossible to compute such a rate. If it is known, however, that the absolute risk (incidence) for males (nonsmokers) age 35 for lung cancer is 0.1/1,000, then the incidence for heavy cigarette smokers is 0.1 × 14, or 1.4/1,000.**

Recommended Readings

1. Mausner, J. S., and Bahn, A. K. 1984. *Epidemiology—An Introductory Text*, second edition, chapter 8. W. B. Saunders Company, Philadelphia.
2. Lilienfeld, A. M., and Lilienfeld, D. E. 1980. *Epidemiology: Foundations*, second edition, chapter 8. Oxford University Press, New York.

Self-Assessment 1

Objectives Covered: 1–7

Best Choice—Select *One* Answer Only

An outbreak of gastritis occurred on a cruise ship. The following data were obtained, shortly after the outbreak, from a questionnaire completed by everyone on board the ship (Table 13).

TABLE 13.

Food	Persons Who Ate Food		Persons Who Did Not Eat	
	Sick	Well	Sick	Well
Herring	200	800	100	900
Chicken	650	350	100	900
Spinach souffle	200	800	500	500
Oysters	300	700	400	600
Chocolate mousse	600	400	450	550

Use these data for questions 1 and 2.

1. What is the most likely infective food on the cruise ship?
   a. herring
   b. chicken
   c. spinach souffle
   d. oysters
   e. chocolate mousse
2. What is the relative risk of developing gastritis for herring consumption?
   a. 0.5
   b. 2.0
   c. 2.3
   d. 8.0
   e. cannot be computed from data given
3. California highway patrol statistics revealed that more accidents occurred to blue cars than to cars of any other color. The inference that, while driving a blue car, one is at higher risk of accident than while driving a car of another color is:
   a. correct
   b. incorrect, because the comparison is not based on rates
   c. incorrect, because no control or comparison group is used
   d. incorrect, because no test of statistical significance has been made
   e. incorrect, because prevalence is used instead of incidence
4. In a study of 500 cases of a disease and 500 controls, the suspected etiological factor is found in 400 of the cases and 100 of the controls. The absolute risk (incidence) of disease in persons with the factor is:
   a. 80%

37

      b. 40%
      c. 16%
      d. 20%
      e. cannot be computed from data given

5. In 1945, 1,000 women were identified who worked in a factory painting radium dials on watches. The incidence of bone cancer in these women up to 1975 was compared to that of 1,000 women who worked as telephone operators in 1945. Twenty of the radium dial workers and four of the telephone operators developed bone cancer between 1945 and 1975. The relative risk of developing bone cancer for radium dial workers is:
      a. 2
      b. 4
      c. 5
      d. 8
      e. cannot be computed from the data given

6. Epidemic refers to:
      a. a disease that has a low rate of occurrence but that is constantly present in a community or region
      b. an attack rate in excess of 10 per 1,000 population
      c. the occurrence of illnesses of similar nature clearly in excess of the normal expectation for that population at that time
      d. diseases of the respiratory system that occur seasonally
      e. the annual case rate per 100,000 population

7. When a new treatment is developed that prevents death but does not produce recovery from a disease, the following will occur:
      a. Prevalence of the disease will decrease.
      b. Incidence of the disease will increase.
      c. Prevalence of the disease will increase.
      d. Incidence of the disease will decrease.
      e. Incidence and prevalence of the disease will decrease.

Regionville is a community of 100,000 persons. During 1960, there were 1,000 deaths from all causes. All cases of tuberculosis have been found, and they total 300—200 males and 100 females. During 1960, there were 60 deaths from tuberculosis, 50 of them in males.
Use the data above for the following five questions (8–12).

8. Crude mortality rate in Regionville is:
      a. 300 per 100,000
      b. 60 per 1,000
      c. 10 per 1,000
      d. 100 per 1,000
      e. cannot be computed from data given

9. The proportionate mortality due to tuberculosis is:
      a. 20%
      b. 30%
      c. 6%
      d. 3%
      e. cannot be computed from the data given

10. The case fatality rate for tuberculosis is:
      a. 6%

b. 20%

c. 2%

d. equal in males and females

e. cannot be computed from data given

11. The cause-specific mortality rate for tuberculosis is:

a. 60 per 100,000

b. 300 per 100,000

c. 200 per 1,000

d. 20%

e. cannot be computed from data given

12. The sex-specific mortality rate for tuberculosis in males is:

a. 0.5 per 1,000

b. 25%

c. greater in males than females

d. 50 per 300

e. cannot be computed from data given

13. Communities P and Q have equal age-adjusted mortality rates. Community P has a lower crude mortality rate than Q. One may conclude that:

a. The two communities have identical age distributions.

b. Diagnosis is more accurate in P than Q.

c. P has an older population than Q.

d. Diagnosis is less accurate in Q than P.

e. P has a younger population than Q.

14. Table 14 shows the sex distribution in three large series of cases of a disease.

TABLE 14.

Series	Male Cases	Female Cases
1	200	100
2	250	50
3	450	150
Total	900	300

The incidence rate of this disease by sex was:

a. twice as great in males as in females

b. three times greater in males than in females

c. five times greater in males than in females

d. from two to five times as great in males as in females

e. cannot be computed from the data given

Table 15 shows data from a large study of bladder cancer and cigarette smoking in Boston.

TABLE 15.

	Bladder Cancer Rates per 100,000 Males
Cigarette smokers	48.0
Nonsmokers	25.4

Use these data for questions 15 and 16.

15. The relative risk of developing bladder cancer for male cigarette smokers compared with male nonsmokers is:
    a. 48.0
    b. 48.0 − 25.4 = 22.6
    c. 48.0/25.4 = 1.89
    d. $\dfrac{48.0 - 25.4}{48.0}$
    e. cannot be computed from the data given
16. The attributable risk of bladder cancer due to cigarette smoking in male cigarette smokers is:
    a. 48.0/25.4 = 1.89
    b. 48.0 − 25.4 = 22.6 per 100,000
    c. 48.0
    d. 48.0/100,000 = 0.00048
    e. cannot be computed from this data

Table 16 shows the total number of persons who ate each of the two specified food items possibly infective with Group A streptococci. Table 17 shows the number of sick persons (e.g., persons with acute sore throats) who ate each of the various specified combinations of the food items.

TABLE 16.   Total Number of Persons Who Ate Each Specified Combination of Food Items

	Ate Pheasant	Did Not Eat Pheasant
Ate caviar	100	100
Did not eat caviar	100	100

TABLE 17.   Number of Sick Persons Who Ate Each Specified Combination of Food Items

	Ate Pheasant	Did Not Eat Pheasant
Ate caviar	50	20
Did not eat caviar	50	25

Use these data for questions 17 and 18.

17. What is the sore throat attack rate in persons who ate both pheasant and caviar?
    a. 50/50
    b. 50/70
    c. 50/75
    d. 50/100
    e. 50/200

18. According to the results shown in Tables 16 and 17, which of the following food items (or combination of food items) is (are) most likely to be the infective item(s):
    a. pheasant only
    b. caviar only
    c. neither pheasant nor caviar
    d. both pheasant and caviar
    e. cannot be calculated from data given

K-type Questions

Key

a	b	c	d	e
1, 2, 3	1 and 3	2 and 4	only 4	all 4
are correct	are correct	are correct	is correct	are correct

19. Examples of prevalence rate(s) include the:
    1. number of episodes of sore throat suffered by a 3-year-old per year
    2. number of new cases of cancer of the prostate per year per 100,000 males
    3. number of cases of diabetes in a high school
    4. total number of cases of multiple sclerosis per 100,000 population per year
20. One hundred twelve persons became ill following, and apparently as a result of, a picnic at which 250 persons were in attendance, including 80 men and 170 women. Of those who became ill, 76 were females and 36 were males.
    1. The sex-specific attack rate for males was 0.32.
    2. The sex-specific attack rate for males was 0.45.
    3. The sex-specific attack rate for females was 0.68.
    4. The overall attack rate was 0.45.

NOTE

$36/112 = 0.32$	$72/112 = 0.68$
$36/250 = 0.14$	$76/250 = 0.30$
$36/80 \ = 0.45$	$76/170 = 0.45$
$122/250 = 0.45$	

5
Biological Variability

Objectives Covered

8. State the purpose of a frequency distribution and cumulative frequency distribution in describing a set of biological measurements.

9. Define a mean, median, mode, and percentile, and describe the features of a distribution that each characterizes.

10. Contrast the features of a normal (Gaussian) distribution with those of skewed distribution.

11. Explain why the mean ± 2 standard deviations is often used to establish the "normal range" and what practical difficulties might be encountered using this procedure in clinical practice.

Study Notes

Variation is inherent in all observed data. Biological measurements, however, are particularly susceptible to variability—from one individual to another, within one individual from one occasion to another, from one observer to another, etc. To assess biological data we need statistical techniques that will help us cope with such variability.

Frequency Distributions

The frequency distribution, as presented in tabular or graphic form, provides a way of organizing a collection of measurements so that we can determine what levels are common and what levels are rare. An example of a frequency distribution table is shown in Table 18. Such a table is developed by grouping the data according to well-defined classes (as shown in the first column of Table 18) and recording the number in each class (as shown in the second column). Thus, the first two columns in Table 18 give the frequency distribution of serum uric acid for the

43

TABLE 18. Distribution of Serum Uric Acid Levels (267 Healthy Male Blood Donors)

Uric acid (mg per 100 ml)	Number of Men	Percent of Total	Cumulative Percent of Total
3.0–3.4	2	0.8	0.8
3.5–3.9	15	5.6	6.4
4.0–4.4	33	12.4	18.7
4.5–4.9	40	15.0	33.7
5.0–5.4	54	20.2	53.9
5.5–5.9	47	17.6	71.5
6.0–6.4	38	14.2	85.8
6.5–6.9	16	6.0	91.8
7.0–7.4	15	5.6	97.4
7.5–7.9	3	1.1	98.5
8.0–8.4	1	0.4	98.9
8.5–8.9	3	1.1	100.0

267 male blood donors. By dividing the number in the class by the total number we obtain the relative frequency, as is shown in the third column of Table 18, expressed as a percent. Notice that this column gives the distribution in a standard form, and it may now be compared with similar distribution data for a collection that differs in size. The fourth column gives the cumulative frequency distribution, which enables us to make a quantitative statement about a given level of the measurement. For example, we can say that about 92% of the individuals in Table 18 have uric acid levels below 7 mg per 100 ml.

A graphic display of the frequency distribution is shown in Figure 7. This graph is called a histogram. A plot of the cumulative frequency

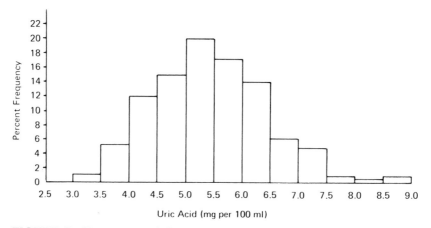

FIGURE 7 Histogram of Serum Uric Acid Distribution in 267 Healthy Males.

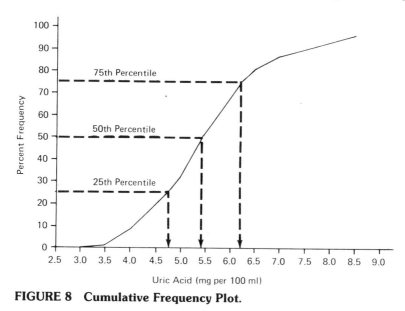

FIGURE 8 Cumulative Frequency Plot.

distribution, as shown in Figure 8, is useful for determining percentiles of the distribution. A percentile is the level of the measurement below which a specified proportion of the distribution falls. For example, from Figure 8 we find that 25% of the distribution falls below a uric acid level of 4.7 mg per 100 ml; 4.7 mg per 100 ml is thus the 25th percentile of that distribution.

Indices of Central Tendency

It is often desirable to have an index that indicates the typical experience for a group. This index would therefore locate the center of the frequency distribution. The mode, median, and mean are three indices of central tendency:

mode = the most frequently occurring observation.

median = that level of the measurement below which half
the observations fall, the 50th percentile

$$\text{mean} = \frac{\text{sum of the observations}}{\text{number of observations}}$$

For any symmetric distribution, the mean, median, and mode will be identical. With a skewed distribution, however, these indices will be arranged as shown in Figure 9, with the mean being the most distorted by extreme observations. The distribution on the right (B) is said to be positively skewed because its longer tail is in the positive direction.

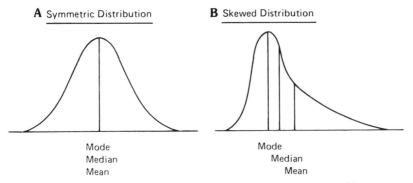

FIGURE 9   **Indices of Central Tendency for Symmetric and Skewed Distributions.**

Indices of Variation

In addition to describing the central tendency it is often desirable to describe the amount of variation present in a collection of measurements. An easy way of doing this is to determine the range, the difference between the highest and the lowest observations. However, because of its mathematical properties, the standard deviation is a much more useful index of variation. The standard deviation is a measure of the average distance of the observations from their mean. Its use in the interpretation of data relates mainly to its role as a parameter of the normal distribution.

The Normal Distribution Curve

The normal (or Gaussian) distribution curve is a theoretical model that has been found to fit many naturally occurring phenomena. To make use of this model we need only have knowledge of the mean and the standard deviation, denoted by μ and σ, respectively. The normal distribution curve has a bell-shaped appearance, symmetric about the mean, with approximately 95% of its relative frequency in the interval $\mu \pm 2\sigma$ (Figure 10). It can also be stated that $\mu \pm \sigma$ includes approximately 68% and $\mu \pm 3\sigma$ includes almost all of the distribution (99.7%).

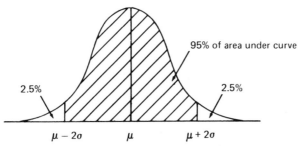

FIGURE 10   **Normal Distribution Curve.**

The Normal Range

It has become common practice in medicine to take as "normal limits" the 2.5th and the 97.5th percentiles of the distribution of the measurement for a healthy population. If it can be assumed that the distribution follows the normal curve, then these limits may be expressed as:

normal limits = mean ± 2 standard deviations

If the distribution is severely skewed, however, then the 2.5th and 97.5th percentiles should be determined in another way. One approach would be to find them on a cumulative frequency plot, such as that shown in Figure 8.

Exercise

Pediatric Serum Cholesterol

Serum cholesterol levels were obtained for 2,033 patients of a pediatrician in Scottsdale, Arizona (Friedman and Goldberg, 1973). This pediatric population was described by the authors as white, middle-class children from a suburban community. Blood samples were obtained by fingerstick at the pediatrician's office. The cumulative distributions shown in Figure 11 summarize the data gathered.

1. **What percentage of the children between seven months and eight years of age had cholesterol levels above 120 mg/dl?**

2. **What is the median cholesterol level for children between the ages of 9 and 19 years?**

3. **What serum cholesterol value would you use to identify children two months of age and under with levels in the highest 5%?**

4. **Which of the children listed below in Table 19 would you classify as abnormal on the basis of serum cholesterol?**

5. **What does Figure 11 tell you about serum cholesterol and its relationship with age?**

6. **From the cumulative distributions given in Figure 11, what can you tell about the shapes of the age-specific frequency distributions for serum cholesterol?**

7. **Why is it better to use the cumulative distribution to obtain normal limits for pediatric serum cholesterol than to use the rule of the mean plus or minus two standard deviations?**

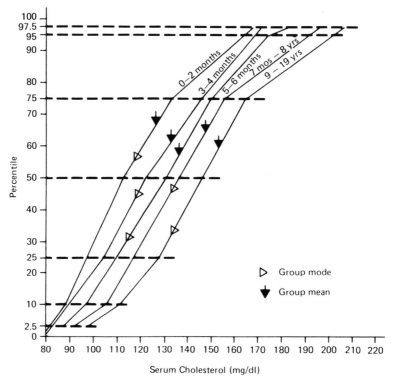

FIGURE 11   Serum Cholesterol Values for Arizona Children.

TABLE 19.

Patient	Age	Serum Cholesterol (mg/dl)
Amy S.	3 years	164
George C.	4 months	183
Kerry H.	3 weeks	150
David H.	5 years	138
Julie K.	12 years	185
Gary M.	1 month	180
Laura V.	7 years	182

Blood Lead and Serum Urea

Raised blood lead concentrations have been investigated for a possible association with renal insufficiency (Campbell et al., 1977). Distributions of blood lead for 54 subjects with raised serum urea and 54 controls matched for age and sex are shown in Figure 12. The mean, median, and mode for each group are shown in Table 20.

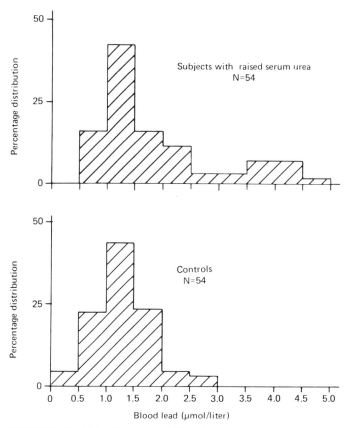

FIGURE 12   Distribution of Blood Lead Levels in People with Raised Serum Urea Concentrations [>6.6 μmol/liter (39.8 mg/100 ml)] and Age and Sex-Matched Controls.

TABLE 20.   Measures of Central Tendency (μmol/liter)

	Subjects with Raised Serum Urea	Controls
Mean	1.73	1.33
Median	1.44	1.31
Mode	1.25	1.25

8. How would you describe the shape of each distribution?

9. What do the measures of central tendency tell you about the shape of the two distributions?

10. When a distribution is of the type shown for subjects with raised urea, the mean is a somewhat misleading indication of the typical level in the group. Why?

Exercise Answers

1. 70%.

2. 145 mg/dl.

3. 160 mg/dl.

4. Taking the 2.5th and 97.5th percentiles as normal limits, we would classify George C. and Gary M. as having abnormal cholesterol levels.

5. There is an increase in cholesterol level with age. This increase is especially pronounced early in life.

6. They are positively skewed. This is evident from the fact that in almost every age group the mean is higher than the median, which in turn is higher than the mode.

7. Since the distributions are skewed, normal limits given by the rule of the mean plus or minus two standard deviations would not represent the 2.5th and 97.5th percentiles.

8. The distribution for subjects with raised urea is positively skewed while that for controls is nearly symmetric.

9. The relationship of the three measures confirms the answer given for 8. For the group with raised serum urea, the mean is appreciably higher than the median, which in turn is higher than the mode. This is characteristic of a positively skewed distribution. All three measures of central tendency are nearly the same for the control group and thus indicate a symmetric distribution.

10. This is because it is distorted by the few subjects with extremely high blood levels. When the distribution is skewed, this effect is not balanced by an equal effect at the other extreme. The median is most often used in this type of situation because it still has a clear interpretation.

Recommended Readings

1. Duncan, R. C., Miller, M. C., and Knapp, R. G. 1983. *Introductory Biostatistics for the Health Sciences,* second edition, chapter 1. John Wiley and Sons, New York.
2. Colton, T. 1974. *Statistics in Medicine,* chapter 2. Little, Brown & Co. Inc., Boston.

References

Campbell, B. C., Beattie, A. D., Moore, M. R., Goldberg, A., and Reid, A. G. 1977. Renal insufficiency associated with excessive lead exposure. Br. Med. J. 482:485.

Friedman, G., and Goldberg, S. J. 1973. Normal serum cholesterol values. JAMA 225:610–612.

6

Probability

Objectives Covered

12. Determine probabilities by using frequency distribution.
13. Explain what is meant by conditional probability.
14. Calculate the probability of complex events by applying the addition and multiplication rules.

Study Notes

The probability of an event is a quantitative expression of the likelihood of its occurrence. Probability is best defined in terms of relative frequency. Thus, the probability (Pr) of an event A is given by:

$$\text{Pr (A)} = \frac{\text{number of times A does occur}}{\text{total number of times A can occur}}$$

Example: In the food poisoning epidemic described in Chapter 1, there were 99 cases of illness among the 158 people who attended the banquet. The probability of illness for a person selected at random is therefore:

$$\text{Pr (illness)} = \frac{99}{158} = 0.63 \text{ or } 63\%$$

Notice that probabilities may be expressed as fractions, decimal fractions, or percentages. Notice also that probabilities, when expressed as decimal fractions, must fall in the range 0 to 1. So that,

Pr (event A does not occur) = 1 − Pr (event A occurs)

Conditional Probability

In the food poisoning example, the probability that a given person became ill was 0.63. However, the probability of illness would have to be modified if we knew what food the person ate. This introduces the idea of conditional probability or, in other words, the probability that A occurs given that B has occurred. The conditional probability for A given B is defined as:

$$Pr (A|B) = \frac{\text{number of times A and B occur jointly}}{\text{number of times B occurs}}$$

Example: Suppose we want to determine the probability of illness for people who ate turkey at the banquet. Expressed as a conditional probability this is:

$$Pr (\text{illness}|\text{ate turkey}) = \frac{\text{number who ate turkey and became ill}}{\text{number who ate turkey}}$$

$$= \frac{97}{133} = 0.73 \text{ or } 73\%$$

If the events A and B are independent, that is, if the occurrence of one does not influence the occurrence of the other, then

$$Pr (A|B) = Pr (A)$$

Complex Events

Events expressed as specified combinations, e.g., A and B, and events expressed as specified alternatives, e.g., A or B, are called complex events.

$Pr (A \text{ and } B)$ = probability that A and B occur jointly

If A and B cannot occur jointly they are called *mutually exclusive* and $Pr (A \text{ and } B) = 0$.

$Pr (A \text{ or } B)$ = probability that A occurs or B occurs or both occur

In other words, $Pr (A \text{ or } B)$ expresses the probability that at least one of the stated alternatives occurs.

There are two rules for combining probabilities that will enable us to deal with complex events more easily. These are the multiplication rule and the addition rule.

The Multiplication Rule

The multiplication rule states that:

$$Pr (A \text{ and } B) = Pr (A|B) Pr (B)$$

So that when A and B are independent, we have:

$$Pr (A \text{ and } B) = Pr (A) Pr (B)$$

Example: Side effects with a certain drug occur in 10% of all patients who take it. A physician has two patients on the drug. What is the probability that both develop side effects?

Here we can assume that the events in question are independent, that is, the occurrence of side effects in one patient does not affect the likelihood of side effects in the other patient. Then,

Pr (both develop side effects) = 0.1 × 0.1 = 0.01 or 1%

The Addition Rule

The addition rule states that:

Pr (A or B) = Pr (A) + Pr (B) − Pr (A and B)

and when A and B are mutually exclusive,

Pr (A or B) = Pr (A) + Pr (B)

Example: What is the probability that at least one of the physician's patients develop side effects?
Notice that the events are not mutually exclusive, and therefore,

Pr (at least one develops side effects) = 0.1 + 0.1 − 0.01

$$= 0.19 \text{ or } 19\%$$

Exercise

Serum Uric Acid Levels in Healthy Males

The frequency distribution of serum uric acid for 267 healthy male adults is given in Table 18 (p. 44). Use this table to answer the following:

1. **What is the probability that a healthy male will have a serum uric acid level in the range of 4.0 to 5.9 mg per 100 ml?**

2. **That he will have a level below 4.0 mg per 100 ml?**

3. **That he will have a level below 4.0 or above 5.9?**

Organ Damage in Hypertensives

A study of end organ damage (Entwisle et al., 1977) was done on hypertensive patients seen at the University of Maryland Hypertension Clinic. Table 21 was compiled from 306 newly identified cases of hypertension and shows evidence of end organ damage classified by severity of hypertension.

4. **What is the probability that a new case of hypertension coming to the clinic will have a history of angina?**

TABLE 21.

		Severity of Hypertension		
		Mild to Moderate	Severe	All
History of angina	+	18	7	25
	−	243	38	281
	all	261	45	306
History of stroke	+	4	1	5
	−	257	44	301
	all	261	45	306
ECG abnormality	+	56	22	78
	−	205	23	228
	all	261	45	306

5. Given that the case has severe hypertension, what is the probability for a history of angina?

6. What is the probability that a new case coming to the clinic will have a normal ECG?

7. Given that the new case of hypertension has a normal ECG, what is the probability that the hypertension is severe?

8. What is the probability that a new case coming to the clinic will have a history of angina and a normal ECG?

9. What is the probability that a new case coming to the clinic will have a history of angina or an abnormal ECG?

10. Two new cases of hypertension come to the clinic on the same day. What is the probability that both have abnormal ECG's?

11. What is the probability that at least one of the two new cases has a history of angina?

Exercise Answers

1. 0.652 or 65.2%.

2. 0.064 or 6.4%.

3. 0.349 or 34.9%.
   Notice that this probability may be determined by using the addition rule:

   Pr (below 4.0) + Pr (above 5.9)

since the two "events" are mutually exclusive, or alternatively, by:

$1 - $ Pr (between 4.0 and 5.9)

4. $25/306 = 0.082$ or 8.2%.

5. $7/45 = 0.156$ or 15.6%.

6. $228/306 = 0.745$ or 74.5%.

7. $23/228 = 0.101$ or 10.1%.

8. We cannot determine this because the "events" are not independent, and therefore:

Pr (angina and normal ECG) $\neq$ Pr (angina) $\times$ Pr (normal ECG)

Notice that if we could get:

Pr (angina|normal ECG)

we could compute the probability needed for the answer. However, this is not possible with the data as provided.

9. It is again impossible to answer this. Since the events are not mutually exclusive, we must use:

Pr (angina or abnormal ECG) =

Pr (angina) + Pr (abnormal ECG)
$$- \text{Pr (angina and abnormal ECG)}$$

We cannot obtain the last term in this expression for the same reasons we could not answer 8.

10. In this case the events are independent, and thus the answer is:

$$\frac{78}{306} \times \frac{78}{306} = 0.065 \text{ or } 6.5\%.$$

11. $0.082 + 0.082 - (0.082)^2 = 0.157$ or 15.7%.

Recommended Readings

1. Duncan, R. C., Miller, M. C., and Knapp, R. G. 1983. *Introductory Biostatistics for the Health Sciences,* second edition, chapter 2. John Wiley and Sons, New York.
2. Colton, T. 1974. *Statistics in Medicine,* chapter 3. Little, Brown & Co. Inc., Boston.

Reference

Entwisle, G., Apostolides, A. Y., Hebel, J. R., and Henderson, M. M. 1977. Target damage in black hypertensives. Circulation 55:792–796.

7

Screening

Objectives Covered

15. Define sensitivity, specificity, and predictive value of a screening test and compute these measures given the necessary data.

16. Describe the selection of screening test criteria with respect to the natural history of the disease in question.

Study Notes

Screening

A screening test is used to separate from a large group of *apparently well* persons those who have a high probability of having the disease under study, so that they may be given a diagnostic work-up and, if diseased, brought to treatment.

Sensitivity and Specificity

These are two ratios used to measure the ability of a screening test to discriminate between individuals who have the disease and those who do not. Sensitivity is the ability to identify correctly those who have the disease. Specificity is the ability to identify correctly those who do not have the disease. These components are determined by comparing the results obtained by the screening test with those derived from some definitive diagnostic procedure. The extent to which the screening results agree with those derived by the more definitive tests provides a measure of sensitivity and specificity.

Sensitivity is the ability of the screening test to give a positive finding when the person tested truly has the disease. It is expressed as a percentage:

$$\frac{\text{persons with the disease detected by screening test}}{\text{total number of persons tested with the disease}} \times 100$$

59

It may seem that sensitivity alone is all one would demand of a test. If it can correctly identify all those with the disease, surely that is sufficient. However, it is necessary that it include as positives only those with the disease. From this restraint stems the concept of specificity.

Specificity is the ability of the test to give a negative finding when the persons tested are free of the disease under study. It is also expressed as a percentage:

$$\frac{\text{persons without the disease who are negative to the screening test}}{\text{total number of persons tested without the disease}} \times 100$$

Sensitivity and specificity of a screening test can be understood more easily by using an example like glaucoma, a disease in which pressure in the eyeball has increased.

The investigator has the problem of setting the cut-off point. Above which particular reading shall the patient be considered by screening to have glaucoma? By studying Figure 13, it is apparent that to detect all glaucomatous eyes (i.e., to attain sensitivity of 100%), the cut-off must be at 22 mm Hg. This level will result in detection of all glaucoma, but at the price of including a considerable number of normal eyes, those in the right-hand tail of the nonglaucomatous distribution, from 22 to 27. This means that the specificity is less than 100%.

Now let us assume that it is desired to exclude all normal eyes, that is, to have a specificity of 100%. Clearly this entails setting the cut-off point at 27, and thus all normals will be excluded, and only glaucomatous eyes detected. However, the price of this will be that some glaucoma is missed, i.e., sensitivity is less than 100%.

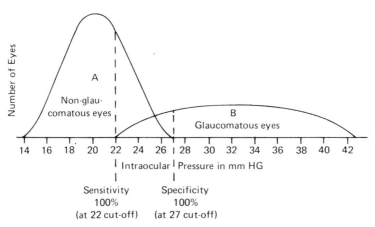

FIGURE 13 Population Distribution of Intraocular Pressures in Glaucomatous and Nonglaucomatous Eyes, Measured by Tonometer (Hypothetical Readings). (Modified from Thorner and Remein, 1961.)

In practice, a compromise is reached and the cut-off point is set as say 24. This means that both the sensitivity and specificity are less than 100%, and both false positives and false negatives will arise, but in small numbers. By studying Figure 13, it is apparent that the sensitivity and specificity cannot both be 100%, while the distributions of well and diseased populations overlap with respect to the variable being measured by the screening test. As the screening test result depends on one cut-off reading only, invariably sensitivity and specificity are related.

Sensitivity may be increased but only at the expense of specificity, and similarly, specificity may be increased but sensitivity decreased in a single test. The cut-off point may be moved in the common territory shared by the well and diseased, and a reciprocal relationship exists between sensitivity and specificity.

The actual setting depends on clinical considerations peculiar to the disease under study. Both the natural history of the disease and the effectiveness of intervention, both early and late, must be known. (If the disease is very rare, sensitivity must be high, or else the few cases present will be missed (PKU is such an example). If the disease has a latent period in development, during which it is asymptomatic, yet maybe detected by a screening test and prognosis improved, screening is very rewarding. If the disease is very lethal and early detection markedly improves prognosis, high sensitivity is necessary. The cancers generally are such examples, in which false positives are tolerable, but false negatives are not. On the other hand, in a prevalent disease, such as diabetes, for which treatment does not markedly alter outcome, specificity must be high, and early cases may be missed but false positives are limited, otherwise the facility is overwhelmed by diagnostic demands on all the positives, but true and false.

Computation of Sensitivity and Specificity

From Table 22 it may be seen that

$$\text{sensitivity} = \frac{a}{a + c}$$

All students always get this right. BUT

TABLE 22.   A General Representation of a Screening Matrix

| Test Result | True Diagnosis | | Total |
	Diseased	Not Diseased	
Positive	a	b	$a + b$
Negative	c	d	$c + d$
Total	$a + c$	$b + d$	$a + b + c + d$

$$\text{specificity} = \frac{d}{b + d}$$

This is tricky, and students sometimes err, making the error of using $b/(b + d)$ by false analogy from sensitivity.

In order to construct such a table from data given in narrative form, it is recommended that you fill in the marginal totals first, before the individual cells.

False Positives and Negatives

The clinician thinks in terms of false positives (b) and false negatives (c). A test that is very sensitive has few false negatives—remember that sensitivity is $a/(a + c)$, so c is small when sensitivity approaches 100%.

A test with a high specificity will have few false positives, since specificity is $d/(d + b)$; therefore, for specificity to approach 100%, b must be small.

Predictive Value of a Positive Test

From Table 22 it will be seen that the proportion of positive tests that are true positives is $a/(a + b)$. This ratio is called the predictive value of a positive test. Physicians are responsible for interpreting for the positive screenees, the meaning of their positive result, and selecting the true positives (a) from the group ($a + b$). The predictive value of a positive test increases with increasing sensitivity and specificity, as might be expected. But if the prevalence of the disease in the population screened increases, the predictive value of a positive test also increases, and the converse is true. High-risk populations are frequently chosen for screening, thus increasing the yield and predictive value of a positive test.

In Table 23 the prevalence of disease is 50%, the sensitivity and specificity are both 50%, and the number screened is 200.

TABLE 23.

Test Result	True Diagnosis		Total
	Disease	*No Disease*	
Positive	50	50	100
Negative	50	50	100
Total	100	100	200

From these data the predictive value of a positive test is 50/100 or 50%.

In Table 24 the prevalence increases to 60%, and the sensitivity and specificity remain at 50%.

TABLE 24.

| Test Result | True Diagnosis | | Total |
	Disease	No Disease	
Positive	60	40	100
Negative	60	40	100
Total	120	80	200

From the data shown the predictive value of a positive test has now increased to 60/100 or 60%.

In Table 25 the prevalence decreases to 40%, and the sensitivity and specificity remain at 50%.

From the data shown the predictive value of a positive test has now decreased to 40/100 or 40%.

TABLE 25.

| Test Result | True Diagnosis | | Total |
	Disease	No Disease	
Positive	40	60	100
Negative	40	60	100
Total	80	120	200

Acceptability

Acceptability of a screening test is a practical consideration. A cervical smear is more acceptable than sigmoidoscopy for example. High-risk groups are frequently identified as target populations for screening programs, yet acceptance is often lowest among those with the greatest probability of disease, the very old or those of low educational attainment, for example.

Exercise

Table 26 shows the results obtained in a screening test for diabetes used on 10,000 persons. The cut-off level employed was 180 mg of blood glucose per 100 ml or above as positive for diabetes.

TABLE 26.

| Test Result | True Diagnosis | | Total |
	Diabetic	Not Diabetic	
Positive	34	20	54
Negative	116	9,830	9,946
Total	150	9,850	10,000

1. **Compute the fractions representing sensitivity, specificity, and predictive value of a positive test.**

When the screening cut-off point was lowered to 130 mg of blood glucose per 100 ml, 98 of 164 persons who then tested positive were among the 9,850 persons judged by diagnostic tests not to have diabetes.

2. **Compute the sensitivity, specificity, and predictive value of a positive test of the test at this cut-off level.**

3. **What effect do you get from lowering the screening cut-off point in terms of false positives, false negatives, and predictive value of a positive test?**

4. **How does this effect the sensitivity and specificity?**

5. **If the cut-off point is set higher than 180 mg of blood glucose per 100 ml,**
   a. **How would you expect this to affect the specificity and sensitivity of the test?**
   b. **What effect will this have on the number of false negatives and false positives?**

6. **In Table 26 assume the prevalence of diabetes increases from 1.5% to 2.0%. Given the same sensitivity and specificity, compute the predictive value of a positive test.**

7. **Your screening facility can process 1,000 persons per week. Assume you are attempting the early detection of a disease with a prevalence of 2%, and that your test has a sensitivity of 95% and a specificity of 90%.**
   a. **How many of a week's screenees will test positive?**
   b. **Of these, how many will be true positives and how many false positives?**
   c. **What is the predictive value of a positive test?**

8. **Suggest a disease for each of the following in which screening leading to early diagnosis has been shown to affect the outcome favorably:**
   a. **for the individual—**
   b. **for the community in general—**

Exercise Answers

1. **Sensitivity = 34/150 or 22.6%.**
   Specificity = 9830/9850 or 99.7%.
   Predictive value of a positive test = 34/54 or 63.0%.

TABLE 27.

| Test Result | True Diagnosis | | Total |
	Diabetic	Nondiabetic	
Positive	66	98	164
Negative	84	9,752	9,836
Total	150	9,850	10,000

2. **The new table at cut-off of 130 mg per 100 ml would be Table 27.**

   Sensitivity = 66/150 or 44%.

   Specificity = 9752/9850 or 99%.

   Predictive value of a positive test = 66/164 or 40%.

3. **Lowering the screening cut-off level of blood sugar that distinguishes between diseased and nondiseased populations will increase the false positives, decrease false negatives, and decrease the predictive value of a positive test.**

4. **Sensitivity will be increased and specificity will be decreased.**

5. a. **If the cut-off is set higher than 180 mg per 100 ml, the specificity will be increased and the sensitivity will be decreased.**

   b. **False negatives increase, false positives decrease.**

6. **Table 26 now becomes Table 28:**

TABLE 28.

| Test Result | True Diagnosis | | Total |
	Diabetic	Nondiabetic	
Positive	45	20	65
Negative	155	9,780	9,935
Total	200	9,800	10,000

   Predictive value of a positive test is $a/(a + b)$ = 45/65 or 69%. Note that the increase in prevalence from 1.5% to 2.0% has increased the predictive value of a positive test.

7. **Out of 1,000 screenees, 20 will have the disease, a prevalence of 2%. Sensitivity of 95% means that $a/(a + c)$ = 95/100. Now, $a + c = 20$, thus $a = 19$, $c = 1$. Specificity of 90% means that $d/(b + d)$ = 90/100. Now, $b + d = 980$, thus $b = 98$, $d = 882$. (See Table 29).**

TABLE 29.

| Screening | Diagnosis | | Total |
	Positive	Negative	
Positive	19	98	117
Negative	1	882	883
Total	20	980	1,000

   a. **An examination of Table 29 indicates that 117 individuals will test positive per week.**

   b. **Of these, 19 will be true positives and 98 will be false positives.**

   c. **Predictive value of a positive test = 19/117 or 16.2%.**

8. a. **Two examples of screening that is beneficial to the individual are:**

   1. **screening for cervical cancer, in all age groups, by cytology**

   2. **screening for breast cancer by mammography, which is beneficial to women over 50 years of age**

   b. **Two examples of screening that is beneficial to the community are:**

   1. **screening for streptococcal infection to prevent rheumatic fever**

   2. **skin testing for tuberculosis**

Recommended Readings

1. Mausner, J. S., and Bahn, A. K. 1984. *Epidemiology—An Introductory Text,* second edition, chapter 9. W. B. Saunders Company, Philadelphia.

2. Lilienfeld, A. M., and Lilienfeld, D. E. 1980. *Epidemiology: Foundations,* second edition, chapter 6. Oxford University Press, New York.

Reference

Thorner, R. M., and Remein, Q. R. 1961. Principles and procedures in the evaluation of screening for disease. Public Health Monograph #67.

8

Sampling

Objectives Covered

17. Use the standard error to compute 95% confidence limits for a mean or a proportion and interpret statements containing confidence limits.

18. Explain sampling bias and describe how random sampling operates to avoid bias in the process of data collection.

19. Distinguish between the standard deviation and the standard error and give one example of the use of each.

Study Notes

The Target Population

The target population is that collection of individuals, items, measurements, etc., about which we want to make inferences. We seldom have data on the entire target population. Instead, we must rely on the information provided by a sample. To make generalizations on the basis of sample results, it is necessary to consider how the sample relates to the target population.

Sampling Error

Sampling error is the difference between the sample result and the population characteristic we seek to estimate. In practice, the sampling error can never be determined because the population characteristic is unknown. However, with appropriate sampling procedures it can be kept small and the investigator can determine the probable limits of its magnitude.

There are two factors that contribute to sampling error:

1. biased selection
2. random variation

67

A biased selection is one from an unrepresentative segment of the population. The error that results cannot be determined. However, even if the sample were chosen in an unbiased way, we would not expect it to be a perfect replica of the population. The sampling error in this case is attributable strictly to chance, and we may think of it as arising from the random variation that would occur from sample to sample (if repeated sampling were done from the same population).

Random Sampling

If the sample is selected in a way that gives each member of the population an equal chance of being chosen, it is a random sample. There are two desirable features of a random sample:

1. It eliminates bias.
2. It enables us to determine the reliability of our result.

For a random sample the only source of sampling error is random variation. Such variation is determined by the heterogeneity of the population and by the size of the sample.

The Standard Error

Just as variability of a measurement is characterized by the standard deviation, the variability of a sample statistic (such as a mean or a proportion) is characterized by the standard error. The smaller the standard error, the more reliable is the statistic. The primary use of the standard error is in constructing confidence intervals.

Confidence Limits

The confidence interval is a useful device for making inferences about the population parameter in which we are interested. In the case of a 95% confidence interval, we can say that there is a 95% chance that the interval will include the population parameter. For reasonably large samples the 95% confidence limits can be expressed as: sample statistic ± 2 standard errors.

Exercise

Cesarean Sections in Baltimore

To determine the proportion of cesarean sections among obstetrical deliveries in Baltimore, a random sample of histories was obtained from two obstetric services: Johns Hopkins Hospital and University Hospital. The rate of cesarean sections for the sample was 20%. Later more complete information revealed that it was not indicative of the general experience throughout the city. Most hospitals in the city were found to have rates ranging from 10% to 12%.

1. **What constitutes the "target population" for this study?**

2. **Why would you regard the sample as biased, even though a random selection of histories was obtained?**

Symptoms of Heart Disease

In an attempt to document the duration between onset of symptoms of heart disease and first attack of myocardial infarction, the experience of 330 patients was recorded (Sigler,1951). These patients had all complained of symptoms to a physician at some time prior to their attack. Their records were used to determine the time from onset of symptoms to attack. The results are given in Table 30.

TABLE 30. Duration Between Onset of Symptoms of Heart Disease and First Attack of Myocardial Infarction

Duration	Number of Cases
1 day	4
2–6 days	12
1–3 weeks	20
1–2 months	28
3–6 months	54
7–11 months	45
1–2 years	50
3 years	23
4 years	22
5 years	16
6 years	12
7 years	8
8 years	12
9 years	4
10 years or more	20
Total	330

3. **How would you define the target population for this study?**

4. **What sorts of cases would tend to be missed from the kind of sample used to measure the duration between onset of symptoms and attack? How would such omissions affect the results?**

5. **Two other methods of determining duration might be considered:**
   a. **Asking patients to recall the onset of symptoms after their attacks;**

b. **Following patients from the time they first report symptoms (including those who never develop an attack).**
Which approach would provide the most accurate information?

6. **What might account for the very long durations given in Table 30?**

Labile Hypertension

A patient who at one time is hypertensive and at another time is normotensive presents a perplexing problem (Julius et al., 1974). A study was made of men who had at least one blood pressure reading over 140 mm Hg systolic or 90 mm Hg diastolic and at least one reading under 140/90 mm Hg for a series of clinic visits. Men of similar age but whose blood pressure was never found to be over 140/90 mm Hg served as a control group. In the hypertensive group, a subgroup was identified consisting of those men whose blood pressure returned to normal when taken at home. It was of particular interest to determine what characteristics of these labile hypertensives might be used to distinguish them from normotensives.

7. **Determine 95% confidence limits for each measure given in Table 31.**

TABLE 31. Clinical Characteristics (Mean or Proportion ± Standard Error) of Subjects in Different Blood Pressure Categories

Characteristic	Normal in Clinic (N = 49)	Borderline in Clinic But Normal at Home (N = 31)
Weight (kg)	70.6 ± 1.5	81.3 ± 1.9
Heart rate (beats per minute)	70.9 ± 1.4	83.1 ± 2.1
Positive family history (%)	24.4 ± 6.1	41.9 ± 8.9

8. **Which characteristics would you regard as having differences too large to be attributed to "sampling error" alone? Why?**

The following rule was used to establish which cases of borderline hypertension could be regarded as having normal readings at home. If the man's home reading was not higher than one standard deviation from the mean home reading among clinical normals (the control group) on both systolic and diastolic blood pressure, he was classified as being normal at home.

9. **What is the rationale for this rule?**

10. **Explain the difference between the use of the standard deviation and the standard error in this problem.**

Exercise Answers

1. All obstetric cases in Baltimore.

2. The sample was restricted by the hospitals used in the study. These are the two teaching hospitals in the city and therefore would be expected to handle an unusually large proportion of difficult cases.

3. To generalize the results in order to make a statement about the duration between symptoms and first attack of myocardial infarction, it seems reasonable to define the target population as all cases of myocardial infarction with prior symptoms.

4. The main source of omission would be unreported symptoms. This could occur for a number of reasons:
   a. death during the time of the first attack
   b. failure of the patient to recognize or report symptoms
   c. faulty recall
   Omission would seem most likely to occur in cases where duration was very short and the patient did not have time to inform a physician. This would lead to an under-reporting of this category.

5. The second approach provides the most accurate information. We would not expect to get as accurate an account of symptoms after the attack has occurred. The patient's state of mind would no doubt influence his ability to recall symptoms as they actually happened. For those cases in which the victim died, we would have to rely on family or friends for such information.

6. The longer the duration, the more likely it is that there were errors in reporting. Such errors might arise by failure to report attacks. It would also seem probable that the longer the duration, the less the symptoms would have to do with heart disease.

7.

TABLE 32. Ninety-Five Percent Confidence Limits on Characteristics of Subjects in Different Blood Pressure Categories

Characteristic	Normal in Clinic	Borderline in Clinic But Normal at Home
Mean weight (kg)	67.6–73.6	77.5–85.1
Mean heart rate (beats per minute)	68.1–73.7	78.9–87.3
Proportion with positive family history (%)	12.2–36.6	24.1–59.7

8. Those for weight and heart rate. For each of these characteristics there is no overlap in the confidence intervals for the two

groups. On the other hand there is considerable overlap in the confidence intervals for family history.

9. Assuming that the distribution of blood pressure readings among those who were established as normotensive at the clinic follows the normal curve, and further assuming that this group is truly normotensive, the rule would lead to misclassification as hypertensives approximately 16% of those who would be really normotensive at home. (See "The Normal Distribution Curve," page 46).

10. The standard deviation expresses variability among individuals and is used therefore to make decisions about individuals. The standard error expresses variability in group statistics and is thus used to make inferences about groups.

Recommended Readings

1. Duncan, R. C., Miller, M. C., and Knapp, R. G. 1983. *Introductory Biostatistics for the Health Sciences,* second edition, chapter 3. John Wiley and Sons, New York.
2. Bourke, G. J., and McGibray, J. 1975. *Interpretation and Uses of Medical Statistics,* second edition, chapter 3. Blackwell Scientific Publications, Oxford.

References

Julius, S., Ellis, C. N., Pascual, A. V., Matice, M., Hansson, L., Hunzor, S. N., and Sandler, L. N. 1974. Home blood pressure determination. JAMA 229:663–666.

Sigler, L. H. 1951. Prognosis of angina pectoris and coronary occlusion. JAMA 146:998–1004.

9

Statistical Significance

Objectives Covered

20. Interpret statements of statistical significance with regard to comparisons of means and frequencies and explain what is meant by a statement such as "$P < 0.05$."

21. Distinguish between the statistical significance of a result and its importance in clinical application.

Study Notes

Interpretation of Comparison Results

The term "statistically significant" is often encountered in scientific literature and yet its meaning is still widely misunderstood. The determination of statistical significance is made by the application of a procedure called a statistical test. Such procedures are useful for interpreting comparison results. For example, suppose that a clinician finds that in a small series of patients the mean response to treatment is greater for Drug A than for Drug B. Obviously the clinician would like to know if the difference he has observed in his small series of patients will hold up for a population of such patients. In other words he wants to know if the observed difference is more than merely "sampling error." This assessment can be made with a statistical test.

To understand better what is meant by statistical significance, let us consider the three possible reasons for the observed Drug A versus Drug B difference:

1. Drug A actually could be superior to Drug B.
2. Some factor that has not been controlled in any way, for example, age of the patients, may account for the difference. (In this case we would have a biased comparison.)
3. Random variation in response may account for the difference.

Only after reasons 2 and 3 have been ruled out as possibilities can we conclude that A is superior to B. To rule out reason 2, we have to have a study design that does not permit any extraneous factors to bias the comparison or else we must deal with the bias statistically, as for example by age-adjustment of rates. To rule out reason 3, we test for statistical significance. If the test shows that the observed difference is too large to be explained by random variation (chance) alone, we state that the difference is statistically significant and thus conclude that Drug A is superior to Drug B.

Significance Tests

Underlying all statistical tests is a "null hypothesis." For tests involving the comparison of two or more groups, the null hypothesis states that there is no difference in population parameters among the groups being compared. In other words, the null hypothesis is consistent with the notion that the observed difference is simply the result of random variation in the data. To decide whether the null hypothesis is to be accepted or rejected, a test statistic is computed and compared with a "critical value" obtained from a set of statistical tables. When the test statistic exceeds the critical value, the null hypothesis is rejected and the difference is declared statistically significant.

Any decision to reject the null hypothesis carries with it a certain risk of being wrong. This risk is called the significance level of the test. If we test at the 5% significance level, we are taking a 5% chance of rejecting the null hypothesis when it is true. Naturally we want the significance level of the test to be small. The 5% significance level is very often used for statistical tests. A statement such as "The difference is statistically significant at the 5% level" means that the null hypothesis was rejected at the 5% significance level.

The *P* Value

Many times the investigator will report the lowest significance level at which the null hypothesis could be rejected. This level is called the *P* value. The *P* value therefore expresses the probability that a difference as large as that we have observed would occur by chance alone. If we see the statement "$P < 0.01$," this means that the probability is very small that random variation alone accounts for the difference, and we are willing to say the result is statistically significant. On the other hand, the statement "$P > 0.10$" implies that chance alone is a viable explanation for the observed difference, and therefore the difference would be referred to as not statistically significant. Although arbitrary, the *P* value 0.05 is almost universally regarded as the cut-off level for statistical significance. This should be taken only as a guideline, however, because, with regard to statistical significance, a result with a P value of 0.051 is almost the same as one with a P value of 0.049.

Sample Size and the Interpretation of Nonsignificance

A statistically significant difference is one that cannot be accounted for by chance alone. The converse is not true, i.e., a difference that is statistically nonsignificant is not necessarily attributable to chance alone. In the case of a nonsignificant difference, the sample size is very important. This is because, with a small sample, the sampling error is apt to be large, and this often leads to a nonsignificant test even when the observed difference is caused by a real effect. In any given instance, however, there is no way to determine whether a nonsignificant difference derives from the small sample size or because the null hypothesis is correct. It is for this reason that a result that is not statistically significant should almost always be regarded as inconclusive rather than an indication of no effect.

Sample size is an important aspect of study design. The investigator should consider how large the sample must be so that a real effect of important magnitude will not be missed because of sampling error. [Sample size determination for two-group comparisons is discussed in Colton (see Recommended Readings).]

Clinical Significance versus Statistical Significance

It is important to remember that a label of statistical significance does not necessarily mean that the difference is significant from the clinician's point of view. With large samples, very small differences that have little or no clinical importance may turn out to be statistically significant. The practical implications of any finding must be judged on grounds other than statistical grounds alone.

Exercise

Proportionate Mortality Among Vinyl-Chloride Workers

In February 1974, four fatal cases of cancer of the liver among men who worked in a polyvinyl chloride polymerization plant were reported (Monson, Peters, and Johnson, 1974). Table 33 gives a proportionate mortality analysis of all deaths from 1947 to 1974 among workers in that plant.

To determine whether or not the excess of cancer deaths could be attributed to chance alone, we do a chi-square test. First, Table 33 is reduced to the form shown in Table 34.

TABLE 33.   Observed and Expected Deaths in Vinyl Chloride Workers[a]

Cause of Death	Observed	Expected	Obs./Exp.
All	161	161.0	1.0
All cancer	41	27.9	1.5
Digestive	13	8.3	1.6
Liver and biliary tract	8	0.7	11.0
Lung	13	7.9	1.6
Brain	5	1.2	4.2
Lymphatic and hemopoietic	5	3.4	1.5
Other cancer	5	7.1	0.7
CNS/vascular	8	9.5	0.8
Circulatory	66	68.6	1.0
External	22	24.3	0.9
Suicide	10	5.3	1.9
All other cases	24	30.5	0.8

[a] Expected numbers based on age/time/cause-specific proportional mortality ratios for U.S. white males.

TABLE 34.

Cause of Death	Observed	Expected
Cancer	41	27.9
All other	120	133.1

Then the chi-square statistic is computed as:

$$\chi^2 = \sum \frac{(\text{observed} - \text{expected})^2}{\text{expected}}$$

$$\chi^2 = \frac{(41 - 27.9)^2}{27.9} + \frac{(120 - 133.1)^2}{133.1} = 7.44$$

This chi-square value has one degree of freedom (df), since only one of the expected numbers can be determined independently of the total number of deaths. To get the P value we now refer to a chi-square table. Table 35 is an abbreviated version of such a table, and from it we see that our computed value of chi-square exceeds that for $P = 0.01$ (for 1 df). We can thus report $P < 0.01$.

TABLE 35.   Abbreviated Table of Chi-Square Corresponding to Selected Values of P

df	0.50	0.10	0.05	0.02	0.01
1	.46	2.71	3.84	5.41	6.63
2	1.39	4.61	5.99	7.82	9.21
3	2.37	6.25	7.82	9.84	11.34
4	3.36	7.78	9.49	11.67	13.28

1. **Is the excess of cancer deaths statistically significant? Why?**

2. **The chi-square value for central nervous system vascular diseases is 0.04 (1 df). Use Table 34 to report a P value. What does the chi-square value tell you about the discrepancy of deaths in this category from the expected number?**

3. **What are the major difficulties with proportionate mortality analysis as a means of revealing the carcinogenic potential of vinyl chloride?**

Oral Contraceptives and Birth Defects

Exposure to exogenous sex steroids during pregnancy was investigated for 108 mothers of children with congenital limb-reduction defects and 108 mothers of normal controls (Janerich, Piper, and Glebatis, 1974). Unintentional use of oral contraceptives early in pregnancy was the primary source of exposure. Of the cases, 15 were found to have been exposed, whereas only 4 of the controls were exposed.

4. **Show, in the form of a 2 × 2 table, the results of this study.**

5. **The chi-square value for the comparisons of rates of exposure among cases and controls was 5.77 (1 df). (See references, for computation of χ^2 from a 2 × 2 table). Use Table 35 to find the corresponding P value. What is your interpretation of the finding?**

Low-Tar/Nicotine Cigarettes

Cigarette consumption was studied (Turner, Sillett, and Ball, 1974) in 10 volunteers smoking cigarettes of progressively lower tar/nicotine content during three consecutive periods of one week each. The subjects recorded the number of cigarettes smoked daily on diary cards. Approximately 30 cigarette butts were collected from each subject during each period. The mean consumption and butt length findings are given in Table 36.

TABLE 36. Cigarette Consumption and Butt Length (Means ± 2 Standard Errors) According to Tar/Nicotine Content

	Tar/Nicotine Content		
	Medium	Low	Very Low
Mean number of cigarettes consumed daily	25.7 ± 6.50	30.9 ± 8.30	29.2 ± 6.20
Mean butt length (mm)	8.84 ± 2.96	7.20 ± 2.82	4.54 ± 2.22

The following remarks are given in the paper:

> When changing from medium to low brands, nine subjects increased their consumption and one reduced slightly, mean consumption rising from 25.7 to 30.9 ($P < 0.01$). There was no significant change in consumption from low to very-low.
>
>   During the medium period the mean butt lengths were 8.84 mm., in the low 7.20 mm., and in the very-low 4.54 mm. The difference between the low and very-low brands was statistically significant ($P < 0.01$).

6. **Did the subjects alter their smoking habits when changing to lower tar/nicotine cigarettes? How? Is there evidence for the assertion that lower tar/nicotine cigarettes cause smokers to consume more tobacco?**

7. **In the study the volunteers were informed of the tar/nicotine content of the cigarettes used during each period. What problems does this introduce? How could the study be done to avoid such problems?**

Propranolol Treatment in Parkinsons' Disease

Propranolol was compared with a placebo in 18 patients with Parkinsons' disease who had been taking stable doses of levodopa for three months or more but who still had tremor (Marsden, Parker, and Rees, 1974). Each patient was given propranolol for a four-week period and a placebo for a similar period but none was aware of the identity of his treatment. A physician, who was also unaware of the treatment plan, scored each patient for total disability, tremor, rigidity, akinesia, posture, handwriting, and circle drawing. Results are given in Table 37.

TABLE 37.   Effects of Propranolol (120 Mg Daily) versus Placebo in 18 Patients with Parkinsons' Disease on Levodopa

	Start Scores[a]	Placebo	Propranolol	Significance[b]
Total disability	27.80	25.70	27.60	N.S.
Tremor	2.67	2.86	2.19	N.S.
Rigidity	4.25	2.92	2.94	N.S.
Akinesia	6.58	6.06	6.75	N.S.
Posture	3.53	4.11	3.86	N.S.
Writing	1.58	1.56	1.28	$P < 0.02$
Circle drawing	1.81	1.94	1.36	$P < 0.02$

[a] A high score indicates severe disability.
[b] Propranolol compared with placebo. N.S., Not significant.

8. **What were the apparent benefits of the propranolol treatment?**

9. **The investigators concluded that the changes that were noted were "not of clinical value and none of these patients have been maintained on propranolol." In view of the fact that certain of**

the findings were statistically significant, what kinds of considerations would lead the investigators to this conclusion?

Exercise Answers

1. Yes. The P value found was less than 0.01, which implies that the probability is very small that the excess is attributable to chance alone. Results having P values of 0.05 or less are usually described as statistically significant.

2. Since χ^2 is less than that given in the table for $P = 0.50$, we report $P > 0.50$. This means that it is quite likely that the small difference between the expected number of deaths and the number observed is due to chance alone.

3. There are two primary problems:
   a. Proportionate mortality analysis does not take into account the absolute risk of dying in the population studied. Thus, it is possible that the mortality rate in vinyl chloride workers is less than that of the United States population, even though there was a disproportionate number of cancer deaths in that group.
   b. A high ratio of observed to expected deaths may be due either to an excess of one cause of death *or to a deficit of another cause.*

4.

TABLE 38.

	Exposed	Not Exposed	Total
Cases	15	93	108
Controls	4	104	108
Total	19	197	216

5. $P < 0.02$.
   The disparity in rates of exposures among cases and controls is too large to attribute to chance alone. Note, however, that this finding does not establish that oral contraceptives cause birth defects, but only that an association exists. (See Chapter 14.)

6. The results indicate that more tobacco was consumed as the subjects moved to lower tar/nicotine content cigarettes. This is reflected by the fact that the mean number smoked was significantly higher for low as compared to medium. And although the number smoked was about the same for low and very low,

the butt length comparison indicates that the subjects smoked more of each cigarette in the case of the very low tar/nicotine content type.

7. The subjects' awareness of the kind of cigarette they were smoking in each period could have influenced their consumption habits. If, for example, they had preconceived notions about the amount of satisfaction they could derive from low tar/nicotine content cigarettes this might have altered the number of cigarettes and the amount of each cigarette that they smoked during the various periods. The study design could have been improved by keeping the subjects "blind" to the tar/nicotine content and by randomizing the order of the three types for each subject.

8. The propranolol improved the patients' performance on the writing and circle-drawing tests. Of the several scores used to assess improvement, only these two showed statistically significant differences for the propranolol-placebo comparison.

9. Even though the drug has produced changes that cannot be attributed to chance, the clinicians had to consider (a) what sort of changes had been produced and (b) how large these changes were. It would seem that the clinicians, in this case, decided that neither the kind of improvement nor its extent warranted continued use of the drug.

Recommended Readings

1. Duncan, R. C., Miller, M. C., and Knapp, R. G. 1983. *Introductory Biostatistics for the Health Sciences*, second edition, chapters 4 and 7. John Wiley and Sons, New York.
2. Colton, T. 1974. *Statistics in Medicine*, chapters 4 and 5. Little, Brown, & Co. Inc., Boston.
3. England, J. M. 1975. *Medical Research*, chapter 1. Churchill Livingstone, Edinburgh.

References

Janerich, D. T., Piper, J. M., and Glebatis, D. M. 1974. Oral contraceptives and congenital limb-reduction defects. N. Engl. J. Med. 291:697–700.

Marsden, C. D., Parker, J. D., and Rees, J. E. 1974. Propranolol in Parkinson's Disease. Letter to the editor. Lancet 2:410.

Monson, R. R., Peters, J. M., and Johnson, M. N. 1974. Proportional mortality among vinyl-chloride workers. Lancet 2:397–398.

Turner, J. A. M., Sillett, R. W., and Ball, K. P. 1974. Some effects of changing to low-tar and low-nicotine cigarettes. Lancet 2:737–739.

10

Correlation

Objectives Covered

22. Interpret the relationship between two variables as displayed on a scattergram, distinguishing between positive, negative, and zero correlation.

23. Explain the information provided by a regression equation as well as that provided by a correlation coefficient.

24. Interpret statements of statistical significance with regard to the correlation coefficient.

Study Notes

Describing Quantitative Relationships

Scientific studies often require a description of the relationship between two variables. Usually in such circumstances we think of one variable as being influenced by the other. It has become conventional to denote the dependent variable, i.e., the one being influenced, by Y and the independent variable by X. We are interested in describing the association between X and Y. To do this we have to measure jointly both X and Y on a series of subjects.

The simplest way of describing the relationship between X and Y is by a graph called a scattergram (Figure 14). To construct a scattergram, the level of Y is plotted against the level of X for each subject. The resulting scattering of points indicates how Y varies with differing levels of X.

Although the scattergram is very useful for gaining a visual impression of the relationship, a more quantitative description is often needed. Two kinds of statistical techniques are used to specify further the relationship between X and Y:

1. regression
2. correlation

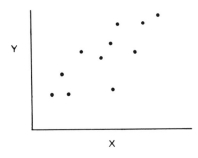

Y

X

FIGURE 14 A Scattergram.

The Regression Equation

The regression approach is appropriate when our main purpose is to develop a predictive model, i.e., a device that will enable us to predict Y given a specified level of X.

Consider the following example. Angiotensin is a substance that raises blood pressure. Suppose we are interested in predicting changes in blood pressure when angiotensin is infused at different rates. We measure the increase in blood pressure at four different infusion rates, and we repeat our measurement four times at each infusion rate. The resulting data are plotted in Figure 15.

The line fitted to the points in Figure 15 gives us a way to predict the expected blood pressure increase at any infusion rate within the range of the graph. This line is found by a procedure called least squares, and it has the best fit in the sense that the sum of the squared deviations of the points from the line is a minimum. The equation of the

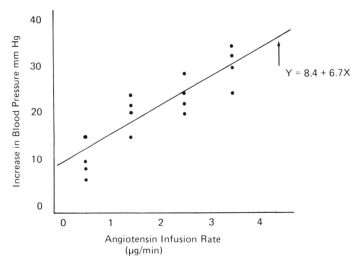

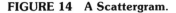

$Y = 8.4 + 6.7X$

FIGURE 15 An Example of a Regression Line Fitted to a Set of Points.

line is called the regression equation. The regression equation has the form: $Y = a + bX$, where a = the intercept, i.e., the value of Y when X is zero, and b = the slope, i.e., the change in Y resulting from a change in X of one unit. The constants a and b are found by the least squares procedure. Of the two, the slope is usually more informative because it shows how much and in which direction Y will vary with changes in X.

By inserting a value for X in the regression equation we can now predict a value for Y. In the example shown in Figure 15, we see there is some variability in the increase in blood pressure at a given infusion rate. We should therefore not expect the regression equation to predict the blood pressure increase exactly. Rather it must be thought of as providing a way of obtaining the average increase in blood pressure for a specified infusion rate.

The Correlation Coefficient

The correlation coefficient, usually denoted by r, is an index of the extent to which two variables are associated. It can take on values between $+1.0$ and -1.0, depending on the strength of the association and whether a positive change in X produces a positive or negative change in Y. A correlation coefficient of zero indicates the two variables are not related (see Figure 16).

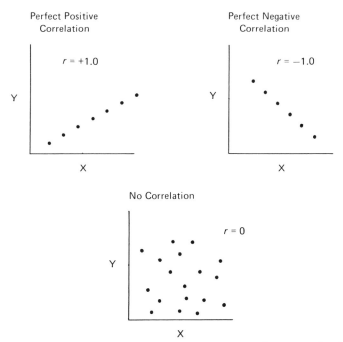

FIGURE 16 **Values for the Correlation Coefficient in Perfect Correlation and No Correlation.**

TABLE 39.

Absolute Value of r	Degree of Association
0.8–1.0	Strong
0.5–0.8	Moderate
0.2–0.5	Weak
0–0.2	Negligible

Table 39 can serve as a general guide to interpreting the magnitude of the correlation coefficient.

Figure 17 shows the correlation between survival time and liver size for 23 children with acute leukemia. In this case there is a moderate degree of association. Notice that the negative correlation coefficient indicates that short survival is associated with large liver size.

As with any statistic, the correlation coefficient is susceptible to sampling error. Thus, our sample may lead us to believe that there is a correlation when none actually exists in the population (see Figure 18).

To rule out the possibility that the correlation we observe is due to chance alone, the hypothesis of no correlation can be tested statistically. The P value in this case is the probability that a correlation coefficient as large or larger than that observed will occur for the sample when no correlation exists in the population. In the example shown in Figure 17,

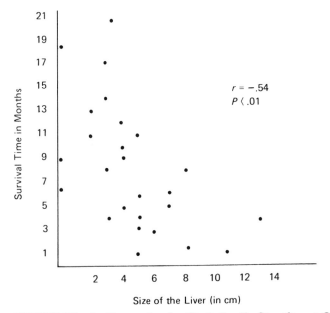

$r = -.54$
$P < .01$

Size of the Liver (in cm)

FIGURE 17   An Example of a Statistically Significant Correlation. (Modified from Halikowski, Armata, and Garwicz, 1966.)

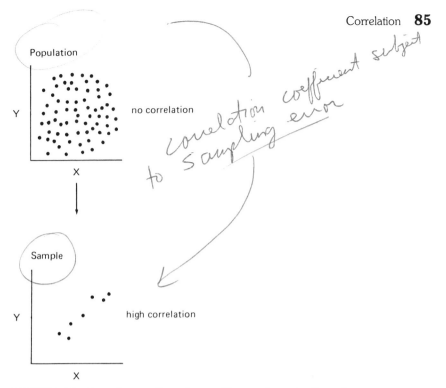

correlation coefficient subject
to sampling error

FIGURE 18   Population Correlation Versus Sample Correlation.

the correlation coefficient is statistically significant at the 1% level, i.e., $P < 0.01$. We may therefore consider the probability to be very slight that the association seen between liver size and survival time is due to chance alone.

Exercise

Hemolytic Disease in Newborn Infants

Studies have challenged the view that newborn infants with Coombs' test-positive hemolytic disease have abnormally high blood volumes (Brans et al., 1974). In this study the investigators attempt to show that when the hematocrit is taken into account, the blood volumes of infants with Coombs' test-positive hemolytic disease are not exceptionally high. Hematocrit, plasma volume, and blood volume were determined for 32 infants with the disease. The observed relationship of plasma volume and blood volume to hematocrit was described in terms of the following regression equations and correlation coefficients:

Plasma volume $= 70.3 - 0.39 \times$ hematocrit

$$r = 0.538, P < 0.005$$

blood volume $= 60.8 + 0.79 \times$ hematocrit

$$r = 0.616, P < 0.001$$

1. **Describe the nature of the association in each case.**

2. **What do the P values indicate?**

3. **Figure 19 shows the blood volumes of the infants with hemolytic disease according to their hematocrit. Also shown is the
   regression of blood volume on hematocrit for normal infants,
   along with the ± one standard deviation range. How do the
   infants with hemolytic disease compare to normal infants with
   regard to blood volume?**

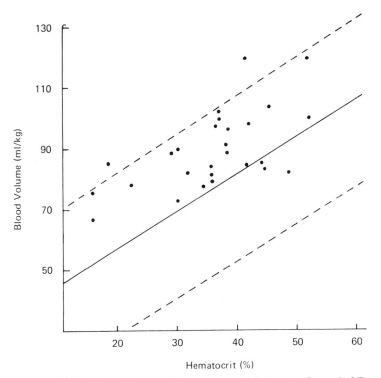

**FIGURE 19   Blood Volume-Hematocrit Relation in Coombs' Test-Positive
Neonates Superimposed Upon the Normal Range (Regression Line ± 1
Standard Deviation for Normal Infants).**

Colon Cancer and Blood Cholesterol

A positive correlation has been observed in international data between
mortality rates for colon cancer and coronary heart disease (Rose et al.,
1974). This relationship is shown in Figure 20.

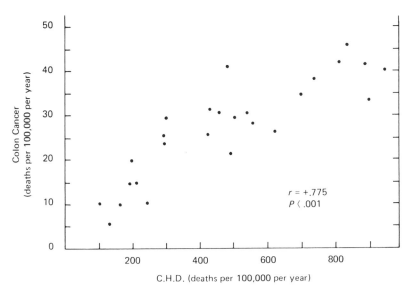

FIGURE 20 National Mortality Rates for Coronary Heart Disease (WHO List, 8th Revision, A.83) and Malignant Growths of the Intestine, Excluding Rectum (WHO List, 8th Revision, A.48), 1969 (Excluding Countries where either Rate was Based on Less than 50 Deaths).

4. What does this sort of association between two apparently unrelated diseases imply?

5. Is it likely that the observed correlation is simply due to chance? Why or why not?

6. Strong positive correlations have also been observed in international data between coronary heart disease and blood cholesterol level. What does this suggest concerning cholesterol and colon cancer?

7. A review of screening tests done in 90 people who subsequently died of colon cancer revealed that the majority had lower cholesterol levels than expected for their age and sex. What sort of association does this finding indicate between cholesterol and colon cancer?

Exercise Answers

1. There is a negative association between hematocrit and blood plasma, i.e., high plasma volumes tend to be found in infants with low hematocrits. A positive association exists between blood volume and hematocrit, i.e., high blood volumes are found in infants with high hematocrits.

2. **In both cases the *P* value is very small, indicating that the probability is small that correlations of the reported magnitude would occur by chance alone.**

3. **Figure 19 shows that although infants with this hemolytic disease tend to have higher blood volumes than the average for normal infants, when hematocrit is taken into account, almost all fall within normal limits.**

4. **An association of this sort suggests shared etiologic factors (common risk factors).**

5. **The small *P* value indicates that this is extremely unlikely.**

6. **This would suggest a positive association between serum cholesterol and colon cancer mortality.**

7. **A negative association. The contradiction we have here in impressions gained from correlations made from international data with those obtained from the study of individuals indicates either:**
   a. **Certain of these associations are artifactual; or**
   b. **The nature of causality is complex.**

Recommended Readings

1. Duncan, R. C., Miller, M. C., and Knapp, R. G. 1983. *Introductory Biostatistics for the Health Sciences,* second edition, chapter 5. John Wiley and Sons, New York.
2. Colton, T. 1974. *Statistics in Medicine,* chapter 6. Little, Brown, & Co. Inc., Boston.
3. Bourke, G. J., and McGibray, J. 1975. *Interpretation and Uses of Medical Statistics,* second edition, chapter 5. Blackwell Scientific Publications, Oxford.

References

Brans, Y. W., Milstead, R. R., Bailey, P. E., and Cassady, G. 1974. Blood volume estimates in Coombs'-test-positive infants. N. Engl. J. Med. 290:1450–1452.

Halikowski, K., Armata, J., and Garwicz, S. 1966. Low-protein purine-free diet in treatment of acute leukaemia in children: Preliminary communication. Br. Med. J. 1:519.

Rose, G., Blackburn, H., Keys, A., Taylor, H. L., Karmel, W. B., Oglesby, P., Reid, D. D., and Stamler, J. 1974. Colon cancer and blood-cholesterol. Lancet 1:181–183.

Self-Assessment 2

Objectives Covered: 8–24

Best Choice—Select *One* Answer Only

A hypertension screening program was carried out in an urban population. Results for diastolic blood pressure among 1,500 males, ages 30 to 69, are shown in Table 40.

TABLE 40.

Diastolic Blood Pressure (mm Hg)	Frequency	Percent
<65	60	4
65–74	270	18
75–84	540	36
85–94	420	28
95–104	150	10
105–115	45	3
>115	15	1
Total	1500	100

Use these data for questions 21–24.

21. Diastolic blood pressure levels of 95 or over were considered to be hypertensive and such cases were referred for further diagnosis. Thus, further testing was initiated for men who:
    a. fell above the 86th percentile
    b. fell above the 97.5th percentile
    c. fell above the 95th percentile
    d. fell below the 14th percentile
    e. fell below the 28th percentile

22. Assuming that the men screened were representative of all men ages 30 to 69 in this urban population, the probability that a man selected at random will have a diastolic pressure of 105 mm Hg or higher is:
    a. 3%
    b. 4%
    c. 14%
    d. 86%
    e. 96%

23. Both the mean and median of the blood pressure distribution are approximately 83 mm Hg and the standard deviation is 12 mm Hg. These indices enable us to deduce each of the following statements *except:*
    a. Approximately 95% of the men have pressure between 59 and 107 mm Hg.
    b. The distribution is nearly symmetric.

89

   c. The 95% confidence limits on the mean for all men, ages 30 to 69, in this population are 59 and 107 mm Hg.

   d. Approximately half of the men have pressures over 83 mm Hg.

   e. The mean is not distorted very much by extremely high pressures in this case.

24. The distribution of diastolic blood pressure for 800 females in this population is nearly symmetric, with about the same standard deviation as that for the males. The mean for the females was 79 mm Hg. Thus we may conclude:

   a. The median will be the same as that for the males.

   b. The normal range will be the same as that for the males.

   c. The standard error of the mean will be the same as that for the males.

   d. There will be a larger proportion of hypertensive females than males.

   e. There will be a smaller proportion of hypertensive females than males.

25. A correlation between two variables measures the degree to which they are:

   a. mutually exclusive

   b. causally related

   c. associated

   d. statistically significant

   e. positively skewed

26. The mean birth weight of first-born infants of 23 women who smoked more than one pack of cigarettes per day during pregnancy was 200 grams lower than that of the first-born infants of 16 women who never smoked. The difference was statistically significant at the 5% level ($P < 0.05$). This means:

   a. Smoking during pregnancy retards fetal growth.

   b. The difference observed between mean birth weights was too large to have occurred by chance alone.

   c. The difference observed between mean birth weights could have easily occurred by chance alone.

   d. The number of patients studied was not sufficient to achieve a conclusive result.

   e. Smoking during pregnancy does not influence fetal growth.

A screening test for breast cancer was administered to 400 women with biopsy-proven breast cancer and to 400 women without breast cancer. The test results were positive for 100 of the proven cases and 50 of the normal women. Use these data for questions 27, 28, and 29.

27. The sensitivity of the test is:

   a. 87%

   b. 67%

   c. 25%

   d. 33%

   e. 12%

28. The specificity of the test is:

   a. 87%

   b. 67%

   c. 25%

   d. 33%

   e. 12%

29. The predictive value of a positive test is:

   a. 87%

   b. 67%

   c. 25%

d. 33%

e. 12%

30. Five percent of pregnant women have evidence of urinary tract infection when they are first seen for prenatal care. Four percent of those who are not found to be infected at the first prenatal visit develop an infection between that time and delivery. The probability that a woman will have urinary tract infection during pregnancy is thus:

a. $0.04 \times 0.95 = 0.038$

b. 0.05

c. $0.04 + 0.05 = 0.09$

d. $0.05 + (0.04)(0.95) = 0.088$

e. $0.04 \times 0.05 = 0.002$

31. People with high levels of plasma high-density lipoprotein (HDL) cholesterol have been found to be at low risk for coronary heart disease. Factors associated with plasma HDL cholesterol were sought in a study of 293 healthy men. Table 41 shows the correlation coefficient and the P value associated with a test of zero correlation for plasma HDL cholesterol and each of the variables listed. All observations were taken at the same time for each of 293 participants.

TABLE 41.

	r	P Value
Plasma triglyceride	−0.42	<0.001
Alcohol intake	0.24	<0.001
Serum glucose	−0.19	<0.001
Body mass index	−0.11	>0.05
Diastolic blood pressure	-0.04	>0.05

Which of the following statements can be made regarding plasma triglyceride?

a. By increasing someone's plasma triglyceride, we can increase his plasma HDL cholesterol level.

b. By reducing someone's plasma triglyceride, we can increase his plasma HDL cholesterol level.

c. High levels of plasma HDL cholesterol tend to be found in men with low plasma triglyceride.

d. Low levels of plasma HDL cholesterol tend to be found in men with low plasma triglyceride.

e. The P value is too small to regard the correlation as anything other than a chance-occurrence.

32. In a study of 50 cases of a disease and 50 controls, it is determined that the difference found with respect to a possible etiologic factor is not statistically significant. One may conclude from this finding that:

a. There is no association of the factor with the disease.

b. The difference may be clinically significant.

c. The difference may be the result of sampling variation.

d. The comparability of cases and controls has been confirmed.

e. Observer or interviewer bias has been eliminated.

33. At age 65, the probability of surviving for the next five years is 0.8 for a white male and 0.9 for a white female. For a married couple who are both white and age 65, the probability that the wife will be a living widow five years later is:

a. 90%

b. 20%

    c. 18%
    d. 10%
    e. 8%

34. The probability that at least one member of the couple will be surviving five years later is:
    a. 98%
    b. 90%
    c. 72%
    d. 28%
    e. 10%

35. A laboratory value with a mean of 18 g/100 ml and a standard deviation of 1.5 implies:
    a. The true value is between 16.5 and 19.5 g/100 ml.
    b. The true value is between 15.0 and 21.0 g/100 ml.
    c. The error is too large for the determination to have any value.
    d. In repeated determinations on the same sample, 95% could be expected to fall between 15.0 and 21.0 g/100 ml.
    e. The true value has a 5% chance of being less than 16.5 or more than 19.5 g/100 ml.

36. Health officials concerned with the dental care needs of children in a low-income community conducted a survey of a random sample of children taken from public school rolls and found that only one in five had seen a dentist within the past five years. However, when a dental clinic was set up for the community, nearly half the children who registered for care had seen a dentist within the past five years. The health officials admitted that the needs of the community were not nearly as great as their sample survey indicated. Select the statement which best describes why you would disagree.
    a. The sample was biased because it did not include children in private schools.
    b. The children are not likely to remember when they last saw a dentist.
    c. The sample was biased because it would tend to exclude the children out of school with serious health problems.
    d. The children who register for dental care are more likely to represent the segment of the community with good health habits.
    e. The sample was probably not large enough.

37. Figure 21 is a scattergram that shows the relationship between systolic blood pressure (BP) and age in 33 women.

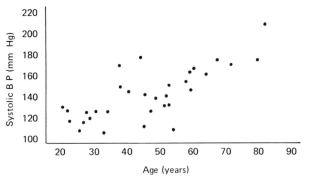

FIGURE 21

Which of the following is the correlation coefficient between systolic blood pressure and age as determined from these data?
a. +1.20
b. −0.22
c. +0.70
d. −0.85
e. 0

K-type Questions

Key

a	b	c	d	e
1, 2, 3	1 and 3	2 and 4	only 4	all 4
are correct	are correct	are correct	is correct	are correct

38. When the distribution of a measurement in a healthy population is severely skewed:
    1. The normal range cannot be determined.
    2. The 2.5th and 97.5th percentiles are best determined from the cumulative distribution.
    3. The 2.5th and 97.5th percentiles are no longer the normal limits.
    4. The mean is distorted by extreme observations.

39. For a random sample of 500 school children in Baltimore City, 27% are found to be susceptible to measles. The standard error of the percentage susceptible is 2%. From this it is correct to conclude:
    1. The probability is 95% that the percentage susceptible for all school children in Baltimore City is between 25% and 29%.
    2. The sample is biased.
    3. The data should be age adjusted.
    4. The probability is 95% that the percentage susceptible for all school children in Baltimore City is between 23% and 31%.

40. Fifty known diabetics, all on insulin, were compared to 50 nondiabetics. The diabetics showed a higher proportion of neurotic responses to a questionnaire ($P < 0.005$). This finding:
    1. could be due to patient characteristic unrelated to diabetes
    2. may be influenced by the effects of insulin
    3. could occur if diabetes caused neurotic responses
    4. is likely to be a chance occurrence

41. In a diabetes detection program the screening level for blood sugar test A is set at 160 mg/100 ml and for test B at 130 mg/100 ml. This would mean that:
    1. The sensitivity of test A is greater than that of test B.
    2. The specificity of test A is greater than that of test B.
    3. The number of false positives is greater with test A than with test B.
    4. The number of false negatives is greater with test A than with test B.

42. As a part of a routine physical examination, uric acid was measured for a 35-year-old male and found to be 7.8 mg per 100 ml. The "normal range" of uric acid for that laboratory is 3.4 to 7.5 mg per 100 ml. If this individual does not display symptoms or signs of gout, the following may be cited as possible explanations:
    1. He is among the small proportion of healthy individuals who yield high serum uric acid readings on a given test.

2. His level is within two standard deviations of the mean for healthy individuals.
3. His gout symptoms have not yet manifested themselves.
4. The departure of his level from the normal range is not statistically significant.

43. The following regression equation was developed from a study of 16 newly diagnosed diabetics who received phenformin for a period of one year:

$$L = -34 + 0.29\ W,$$

where L is the patient's weight loss one year after therapy began, and W is the patient's initial weight. On the basis of this information we may conclude:
1. All patients lost at least 34 pounds during the first year of therapy.
2. The regression line fitted to a scattergram of weight lost versus initial weight would have a positive slope.
3. The correlation between weight loss and initial weight is positive and very strong.
4. Patients who weighed more than others at the beginning of therapy lost more weight, on the average, during the first year of therapy.

44. A report of a clinical trial of a new drug versus a placebo noted that the new drug gave a higher proportion of success than did the placebo. The report ended with the statement: $\chi^2 = 4.72, P < 0.05$. In light of this information, we may conclude:
1. Fewer than one in 20 will fail to benefit from the drug.
2. The chance that an individual patient will fail to benefit is less than 0.05.
3. If the drug were effective, the probability of the reported finding is less than one in 20.
4. If the drug were ineffective, the probability of the reported finding is less than 0.05.

45. In a study designed to determine the five-year incidence of hypertension in an inner-city community, a 15% random sample of normotensives is selected for follow-up. Which of the following should be done to avoid a biased estimate of incidence of hypertension in the community?
1. Repeated attempts should be made to contact members of the sample who are difficult to reach for follow-up measurements.
2. Death certificates should be examined for members of the sample who died in the five-year period to determine if their deaths were hypertension related.
3. Efforts should be made to locate members of the sample who move out of the community during the five-year period so that their blood pressure status can be determined.
4. Members of the sample who refused to have their blood pressure taken during the follow-up should be replaced by residents who are more cooperative.

11

Retrospective Studies

Objectives Covered

25. Distinguish between experimental and observational studies.
26. Describe the following type of epidemiologic study:
  a. case-control

Study Notes

Experimental and Observational Studies

Experimental studies are the most easily recognizable because in these the investigator has control of some factor that, when varied, may be associated with different outcomes. Classically, this is usually seen in animal studies in which diet, for example, may be controlled and reproductive indices and growth rates measured. In human studies, however, ethical considerations limit the applicability of the experimental method, and the investigator must use the observational approach. Here, no manipulation is attempted, but differing outcomes are observed under natural conditions and related to differing exposures. People have some attribute, such as blood type A, or exposure, such as oral contraceptives usage, and the development of disease in the group with the attribute is compared to that in the group without. The difficulty is that the observed groups may differ in other ways in addition to the attribute in question, which possibility confounds the comparison.

In order to label a study as experimental or observational, look for the hallmark of investigator control. If present, it signifies an experimental study. The remainder, the majority in human studies, are observational.

95

Sequence of Investigation for Etiology of Disease

First, the clinician makes an observation regarding cause, based on his or her experience. For example, in 1941 Gregg, an Australian opthalmologist, reported a new syndrome of congenital cataract, and linked it to rubella in the mother during the pregnancy. Clinical observations such as this provide leads from which hypotheses are formulated. These hypotheses are then tested in sequence by retrospective (case-control) studies, and if these are positive, by prospective (cohort) studies. Risk factors are then identified and an intervention trial may be designed to ascertain if modification of such factors in patients is followed by reduction in amount of disease.

Study Design

The majority of epidemiologic studies have to complete the 2 × 2 table shown in Table 42.

TABLE 42.

		Disease	
		Present	Absent
Exposure	Present	a	b
	Absent	c	d

"Exposure" is used here in a general sense, including the presence of an attribute such as hypertension, or any suspect etiological factor. "Disease" is used here, but it can include any outcome, such as survival.

If the approach is retrospective, the investigator starts with $a + c$ cases (Table 42). A comparison group of $b + d$ controls (Table 42) is then selected and the position shown in Table 43 is reached. The participants are then retrospectively assigned to the exposure rows, so the 2 × 2 table is then completed (see Table 42). Analysis is then performed by comparing the exposure rates between the case and control groups:

$$\text{exposure rate among cases} = \frac{a}{a + c}$$

$$\text{exposure rate among controls} = \frac{b}{b + d}$$

When the design is prospective, however, the investigator starts with the row total $a + b$ (the exposed group), and the row total $c + d$ (the nonexposed group), and the position shown in Table 44 is reached. The participants are then followed forward, and they eventually fall into the disease or nondisease columns, so the 2 × 2 table is completed prospec-

TABLE 43.

		Disease	
		Present	*Absent*
Exposure	Present	?	?
	Absent	?	?
	Total	$a + c$	$b + d$

tively (see Table 42). Analysis is then performed by comparing the rate of disease occurrence (incidence) between the exposed and nonexposed groups:

$$\text{incidence in the exposed group} = \frac{a}{a + b}$$

$$\text{incidence in the non-exposed group} = \frac{c}{c + d}$$

TABLE 44.

		Disease		
		Present	*Absent*	Totals
Exposure	Present	?	?	$a + b$
	Absent	?	?	$c + d$

The advantage of the retrospective design is that it may be used to study a rare disease, for cases of a rare disease may be retrospectively collected from a group of large hospitals and compared with controls free of the disease. The prospective design, by contrast, entails assembling a study cohort, free of the disease under consideration, and following them forward in time so as to observe the development of the disease among some of their members. With a rare disease, however, the number of cases would be very small. Further, the retrospective study yields a result in a relatively short time. This may be important if the outcome is a suspected pathology resulting from drug exposure. The price to be paid for these two advantages is that the probability of bias is greater in a retrospective study than in the prospective approach.

Bias

Bias is systematic error, resulting in over- or underestimation of the strength of the association. The validity of any study depends on the accuracy with which the subjects are assigned to the four categories, *a, b, c,* and *d* (Table 42). Misclassification may occur because of over- or underdiagnosis. If a disease entity is well defined, such as cancer of the lung, the diagnosis being uniform and established, the majority of cases coming to medical attention, and there is little selectivity by physicians in hospitalizing the patient, misclassification is minimal. Thromboembolic phenomena present a contrast. The disease is difficult to diagnose, it may present as a complication of another medical or surgical condition, and criteria are not uniform. Also the presence or absence of exposure may influence the management. If a physician is faced with a young woman, known to be on oral contraceptives, presenting with leg pain, she may be hospitalized more readily than another similar patient not on oral contraceptives. The control group is represented by the participants in the column total $b + d$. It is necessary to ensure the disease is absent in this group, which may be simple in the case of lung cancer, but less certainty prevails with thromboembolic disease.

The sample of cases studied may not represent the entire spectrum of the disease. Hospitalized cases may exclude mild cases and those who die prior to admission. Coronary heart disease is such an example.

The design in Table 42 also assumes that the exposure is present or absent, both categories, of course, being mutually exclusive. The exposure may be difficult to define and measure, e.g., type A personality, or difficult to recall, as in drug use. Furthermore, the exposure may be intermittently present, for example, oral contraceptive use. Thus, the row total $a + b$ may over- or underrepresent the exposure in the sample. If the information sought is unchanging and usually available, such as blood group, bias may be minimal. In a more usual case, the needed information is not available and is sought by interview or questionnaire. The recall of events in the distant past may be inaccurate, or the information supplied by the informant may be biased.

Selective recall may occur among the cases, as they necessarily know they have the disease, and may already associate it with exposure. The interviewer, being aware of the identity of cases and controls, may unconsciously probe more among the cases, seeking a positive association. To minimize bias from this source, the interviewer ideally should be unaware of which participant is a case or control, but this is difficult to achieve in retrospective studies.

Bias may occur in the selection of controls, particularly if hospitalized patients are used, as is frequently the case. It is essential that the control group be as much like the diseased group as possible, yet also similar to the general population in distribution of the exposure if the results are to be extended to the general population. The hospitalized controls may contain an unrepresentative proportion of a particular attribute, hypertensives and smokers, for example.

Matching

The comparison between cases and controls may reveal a difference in exposure rates, and the development of disease may be ascribed to this difference, provided the two groups are otherwise comparable. In order to attain such comparability, they are frequently matched for characteristics known to influence the distribution of exposure. Age is frequently such a factor; therefore, in order to eliminate this effect from the comparison, the controls are matched to the cases for age. Socioeconomic status (SES), because it influences environmental hazards and life styles, frequently affects exposure rates and therefore is used to match cases with controls. It should be emphasized that when a variable is used for matching, its etiologic role cannot be investigated because cases and controls are then automatically similar with respect to that characteristic.

Testing a Hypothesis

Let our hypothesis be that smoking is associated with lung cancer. Take 100 cases of lung cancer, and then choose 100 controls free of lung cancer from the general population, similar with regard to age, sex, and SES; the resulting scale is shown in balance in Figure 22a. Now ascertain the smoking habits of the two groups; Figure 22b depicts the resulting imbalance. You have shown an *association* between smoking and lung cancer.

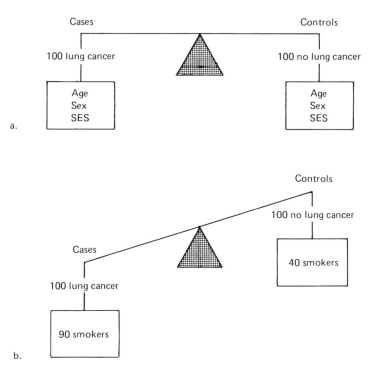

FIGURE 22 Cases and Controls are Similar with Regard to Age, Sex, and SES (a) but Differ in Smoking Habits (b).

Analysis of Results

At the beginning of our study, the 2 × 2 is only completed to the degree shown in Table 45.

TABLE 45.

	Cases	Controls
Smokers	?	?
Nonsmokers	?	?
Total	100	100

During the study we retrospectively determine the number of smokers and nonsmokers in both the case and control group. Thus, we find a, b, c, and d for the 2 × 2 table, as shown in Table 46.

TABLE 46.

	Cases	Controls
Smokers	90	40
Nonsmokers	10	60
Total	100	100

Now we compare exposure rates for cases and controls, thus:

$$\text{case exposure rate: } \frac{a}{a + c} = \frac{90}{100} \text{ or } 90\%$$

$$\text{control exposure rate: } \frac{b}{b + d} = \frac{40}{100} \text{ or } 40\%$$

$$P < 0.001$$

Statistical significance attached to the result is determined with a chi-square test, as described earlier.

Odds Ratio and Estimation of Relative Risk

Because of the retrospective nature of the study, we cannot derive incidence for either the smokers or the nonsmokers. However, it is possible to estimate relative risk provided two assumptions are valid:

1. The disease has low incidence in the general population. (This is true for the majority of chronic diseases.)
2. The control group is representative of the general population with respect to the frequency of the attribute.

Under such circumstances a statistic called the odds ratio gives a close approximation to the relative risk:

$$\text{odds ratio} = \frac{ad}{bc}$$

In the example the odds ratio is:

$$\frac{90 \times 60}{40 \times 10} = 13.5$$

and provides an estimate of the relative risk for smokers.

Exercise

In case-control studies:

1. a. **Your cases are 100 women with breast cancer. What is the essential prerequisite of the control group?**
   b. **Your hypothesis is that young age at first pregnancy is protective against breast cancer—should you match for SES in cases and controls? Give your reasons.**
   c. **Is it possible to test the hypothesis that breast cancer rates are higher in single women than in married, using the same 100 cases and 100 controls?**
   d. **Suppose you found that 80% of the breast cancer cases were married, does this demonstrate that being married increases the risk of developing breast cancer?**
   e. **Assume that 90% of the control group are married. Estimate the relative risk of breast cancer for single women.**

2. **Your hypothesis is that alcoholics have an increased incidence of fatal automobile accidents. Design a case-control study to test this hypothesis using the following headings:**
   a. **Diagnosis of cases—difficult or not? Where would you find cases?**
   b. **Name a suitable population from which to choose controls.**
   c. **List matching characteristics for controls.**
   d. **What characteristic must you now determine for each study member?**
   e. **What difficulties might be encountered in determining this characteristic?**

Exercise Answers

1. a. **The controls should be free of breast cancer.**
   b. **Yes, SES affects age at first pregnancy, so if you demonstrate an association, it may be due to SES unless you matched for it.**
   c. **Yes, we may ascertain the proportion of single women in each group.**

    d. No, we need to compare the frequency of marriage in the control group.

    e.

TABLE 47.

	Cases	Controls
Single	20	10
Married	80	90
Total	100	100

$$\textbf{Odds ratio = estimate of relative risk} = \frac{20 \times 90}{10 \times 80} = 2.25.$$

2. **a. Little difficulty in diagnosis of death from automobile accidents. You can find cases in the medical examiner's office or in police records and highway death statistics.**

    b. From other automobile drivers in the state who have not had fatal accidents. Notice that the controls should be drivers, as alcoholics may be overrepresented in the nondriving population, having lost their licenses.

    c. Age, sex, SES (any characteristic that you think relevant to fatal automobile accidents may be used as a matching characteristic, but NOT alcohol usage).

    d. Some measure of alcohol usage.

    e. Alcohol usage for deceased drivers might be difficult to ascertain, and control drivers may give false information on this point.

Recommended Readings

1. Mausner, J. S., and Bahn, A. K. 1984. *Epidemiology—An Introductory Text*, second edition, chapter 8. W. B. Saunders Company, Philadelphia.
2. Lilienfeld, A. M., and Lilienfeld, D. E. 1980. *Epidemiology: Foundations*, second edition, chapter 8. Oxford University Press, New York.

Reference

Gregg, N. M. 1941. Congenital cataract following German measles in the mother. Trans. Ophthalmol. Soc. Aust. 3:35.

12

Prospective Studies

Objectives Covered

26. Describe the following types of epidemiologic studies:
   b. prospective
   c. cross-sectional
27. Define cohort and recognize a cohort effect when interpreting cross-sectional data.

Study Notes

Four different descriptive terms are used for prospective studies: cohort, incidence, prospective, and longitudinal. The four names of this type of study each emphasize a different aspect of the study. *Cohort* refers to the study group. *Incidence* refers to the fact that incidence (absolute risk) may be derived from this type of study—whereas it may not from a case-control study. *Prospective* refers to the fact that the study group is followed forward in time to the future, and is contrasted to *retrospective*, which goes back in time to the past. *Longitudinal* refers to the fact that study participants, once identified, are followed individually forward throughout the course of the study.

In a retrospective (case-control) study, all of the relevant events (disease and exposure) have already occurred when the study is started. In a prospective study the exposure has occurred, but the disease has not.

As can be seen from studying Figure 23, the investigator first assembles a group of volunteers (cohort) and examines them to make certain they are free of the disease in question at the start of the study. Numerous items of information (variables) are then collected, such as demographic data, including occupational, medical, and social status. These variables must obviously include those that eventually prove rele-

103

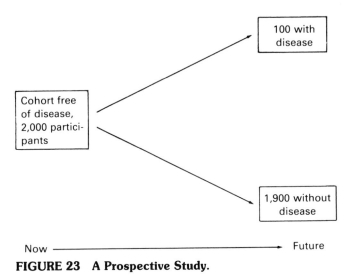

FIGURE 23   A Prospective Study.

vant to the etiology of the disease. The prospective design, by its very nature, avoids two of the most potent causes of bias in the retrospective approach, namely the selection of controls and bias in ascertaining exposure. The control group in this case consists of those persons without the suspected exposure and is thus not selected by the investigator. Because the exposure must necessarily occur prior to the development of the disease, there is less bias in ascertaining exposure: neither the observer nor the participants are prejudiced by prior knowledge of who has the disease and who has not.

One of the major limitations of the prospective approach stems from the fact that participants must all volunteer, and they must return at regular intervals to be examined for development of the disease and for variations in the exposure and other factors being monitored. Employed groups are frequently chosen because they are relatively easy to follow for some years. Railroad or government employees may be used, and such people differ both from the unemployed and from those in less secure occupations, e.g., salespeople, brokers, and many in entrepreneurial fields. The latter group may be exposed to more and different stresses, and the lure of the occupation may cause self-selection among its practitioners. The results of a study of an employed group are only strictly applicable to other similarly employed groups and are not necessarily generalizable to the population at large.

Thus, a cohort of healthy individuals is brought under observation and is classified with respect to the characteristics of interest (variable) to the investigator. If the rate of development of coronary heart disease (incidence) is to be studied, the cohort members are first examined to exclude those with preexisting coronary heart disease. They (the cohort) are then kept under observation of a kind sufficient to identify those who develop the condition that is under study (in our example, coronary heart disease). In this way incidence rates for the disease may be developed for persons who are exposed and those who are not. To take another example, we might establish incidence rates of lung cancer over a 10-year period among persons categorized as smokers at the start of the period and contrast them with rates among nonsmokers.

Persons Lost to Follow-up

In prospective studies a small number of the group will be lost as the study ages year by year. It is generally assumed that the participants lost to follow-up have the same incidence of disease and the same outcome as those who remain under observation. This assumption may be fallacious. Those who develop the disease may have migrated in order to get the disease treated, or they may move less than those remaining free of the disease, thus overstating the incidence of the disease in the latter event and understanding it in the former. Attrition must be held to an acceptable minimum, in order for the conclusions from the study to remain valid. It is this constraint (attrition) that influences investigators to follow employed groups in preference to general population samples.

Analysis of Results

Consider a cohort of 2,000 persons of which 800 are smokers and 1,200 are nonsmokers. At the beginning of the study our 2 × 2 table is Table 48.

TABLE 48.

	Lung Cancer	No Lung Cancer	Totals
Smokers	a	b	800
Nonsmokers	c	d	1,200
Totals	$a + c$	$b + d$	2,000

The entire cohort is followed for 20 years, and 100 develop lung cancer, of whom 90 are smokers and 10 are not. In Table 49 now we complete the 2 × 2 table.

TABLE 49.

	Lung Cancer	No Lung Cancer	Totals
Smokers	90	710	800
Nonsmokers	10	1,190	1,200
Totals	100	1,900	2,000

We next compare incidence rates for smokers and nonsmokers:

$$\text{smokers:} \frac{a}{a+b} = \frac{90}{800} = 112.5 \text{ per } 1000$$

$$\text{nonsmokers:} \frac{c}{c+d} = \frac{10}{1200} = 8.3 \text{ per } 1000$$

$$P < 0.001$$

Here again we determine statistical significance using a chi-square test.

Computation of Relative Risk

In a prospective study we are able to determine incidence rates directly in those exposed and those not. Thus, we calculate the relative risk as the ratio of the two incidences:

$$\text{relative risk} = \frac{a/(a+b)}{c/(c+d)}$$

In the example the relative risk is

$$\frac{90/800}{10/1200} = 13.5$$

Comparison with Retrospective Studies (Table 50)

TABLE 50. Retrospective and Prospective Studies: Advantages and Disadvantages

Retrospective	Prospective
+ Short study time	− Long time required
+ Relatively inexpensive	− Very costly
+ Suitable for rare disease	− Relatively common diseases only
+ Ethical problems minimal	− Ethical problems may be considerable and influence study design
− Control group has bias in selection	+ Control group less susceptible to bias
+ Subjects need not volunteer (chart audit)	− Volunteers needed—results may not be generalized
− Biased recall	+ No recall necessary
+ Small number of subjects	− Large number of subjects
+ No attrition problems	− Attrition problems
− Cannot determine incidence	+ Incidence determined
− Relative risk approximate	+ Relative risk accurate

Retrospective and prospective studies are not competing methods. Clinical observation or a prevalence survey (cross-sectional study) may provide the first suggestion of an association between exposure to a factor and development of disease. This hypothesis is then tested by means of a retrospective study. If the association is confirmed, a prospective study is often done.

Cohort

A cohort is a group of persons who share a common experience within a defined time period.

A birth cohort is the commonest example seen, but a cohort might be all those of one graduating class or survivors of myocardial infarction in one particular year. By following such a group forward for disease outcome, it is possible to distinguish between the influence of aging and underlying secular trends in the disease.

It is important to recognize a possible cohort effect in cross-sectional data, particularly in interpretation of survey data, which are commonly presented. An apparent trend shown in the cross-sectional data may be due to the cohort effect. For example, a study of a retrospective sample of general practitioners in North Carolina included, among other things, information on the number of medical journals subscribed to annually (see Table 51). The inference that, as they grow older, general practitioners in North Carolina read fewer journals is incorrect because a cohort effect is operating. The trend toward reading fewer journals after age 50 is due to the presence, in that age group, of a cohort of physicians trained when fewer journals were published. In order to determine how reading habits vary with age, it is necessary to follow physicians' reading habits as they age.

Cross-Sectional Studies

These studies determine prevalence, not incidence. Their use is largely in prevalence determinations rather than in etiological investigation. For example, to ascertain the prevalence of hypertension in Baltimore City, the blood pressure of a sample of adult residents was taken in 1983. Other items of information gathered during the survey included age, sex, race, and occupation. Thus, we can determine how the prevalence of the condition is related to the variables measured. Such a study tells us

TABLE 51.

Age Group of Physicians	Number of Physicians	Mean Number of Journals Purchased
Under 30	5	4.5
30–39	34	4.2
40–49	27	4.6
50–59	21	3.6
60 and over	6	2.3

about the distribution of a disease in the population, rather than its etiology. However, distribution patterns may suggest etiological hypotheses that can be tested by case-control studies and later by prospective studies.

Exercise

1. **A cross-sectional study in 1976 revealed that the prevalence of oral contraceptive (o.c.) use varied with age, as shown in Table 52.**

TABLE 52.

Age	Prevalence of O.C. Use
15–19	15%
20–24	25%
25–29	22%
30–34	15%
35–39	7%
40–44	3%

The inference from these data that, as women grow older, they cease using oral contraceptives is:
a. **correct**
b. **incorrect because a rate is necessary to support the observation**
c. **incorrect because no control or comparison group is used**
d. **incorrect because a cohort effect may be operating**
e. **incorrect because prevalence is used whereas incidence is necessary**

For questions 2, 3, 4, 5, and 6, assign the studies described to one of the types listed below:
A. uncontrolled observation
B. cross-sectional or prevalence study
C. experiment
D. prospective study
E. retrospective or case-control study

_____ 2. **Four rats in one cage were found dead at the university animal colony. In the adjacent cage, one rat convulsed and died, two rats became ill but survived, and one rat was ill. The veterinarian declared that an epizootic was present (epizootic—epidemic in animals).**

_____ 3. **Fifteen hundred adult males working for Lockheed Aircraft were initially examined in 1951 and were classified by diagnosis criteria for coronary artery disease. Every three years they have been examined for new cases of this disease; attack rates in different subgroups have been computed annually.**

_____ 4. **A random sample of middle-age sedentary males was selected from four census tracts, and each man was examined for coronary artery disease. All those having the disease were excluded from the study. All others were randomly assigned to either an exercise group, which followed a two-year program of systematic exercise, or to a control group, which had no exercise program. Both groups were observed semiannually for any difference in incidence of coronary artery disease.**

_____ 5. **One hundred persons with infectious hepatitis and 100 matched neighborhood well controls were questioned regarding a history of eating raw clams or oysters within the preceding three months.**

_____ 6. **Questionnaires were mailed to every 10th person listed in the city telephone directory. Each person was asked to list age, sex, smoking habits, and respiratory symptoms during the preceding seven days. Over 90% of the questionnaires were completed and returned. Prevalence rates of upper respiratory symptoms were determined from the response.**

Adenocarcinoma of the Vagina

Adenocarcinoma of the vagina in young women had rarely been recorded before the report of eight cases treated at the Vincent Memorial Hospital, Boston, between 1966 and 1969. The unusual occurrence of this tumor in eight patients born in New England hospitals between 1946 and 1951 led to an investigation. Attention was particularly directed at a history of maternal ingestion of estrogens during the pregnancy that resulted in the patient with vaginal adenocarcinoma.

7. **What type of epidemiologic study would be appropriate for this problem and why?**

Exercise Answers

1. d. **The inference may be true, but it cannot be derived from this cross-sectional data because of a possible cohort effect operating. It is necessary to follow a cohort forward in time and record the individuals' o.c. usage.**

2. **A. uncontrolled observation**
3. **D. prospective study**
4. **C. experiment**
5. **E. retrospective or case-control study**
6. **B. cross-sectional or prevalence study**
7. **A retrospective (case-control) study would be appropriate because 1) the disease is very rare; 2) the diagnostic accuracy is high; 3) cases would not be missed; 4) the history of exposure to the suspected causative factor could be reliably obtained by history and/or records; and 5) relative risk can be estimated.**

Recommended Readings

1. Mausner, J. S., and Bahn, A. K. 1984. *Epidemiology—An Introductory Text,* second edition, chapter 8. W. B. Saunders Company, Philadelphia.
2. Lilienfeld, A. M., and Lilienfeld, D. E. 1980. *Epidemiology: Foundations,* second edition, chapter 9. Oxford University Press, New York.

13

Randomized Clinical Trials

Objective Covered

26. Describe the following type of epidemiologic study:
d. randomized clinical trials

Study Notes

The experiment is the strongest weapon in the scientific armamentarium to test a hypothesis. In the physical sciences the experimental method is ordinarily chosen. Animal experiments are common in biology, but when human subjects are involved, opportunities for experimentation are limited.

The purpose of the retrospective and prospective studies described in the two previous chapters has been to identify the etiology of disease. The experimental intervention studies now described usually have a different primary purpose, namely to determine which is superior among competing treatments (see Figure 24). This involves the randomization of patients to various treatment groups, and it is this characteristic (randomization) that is the hallmark and is "pathognomic" of clinical trials.

These studies are prospective in nature, i.e., the entire group of participants must be followed forward and monitored for outcome. In addition, these studies have the distinction of being experimental, that is, the investigator manipulates or intervenes with one group and withholds such treatment from another group. This is in contrast to the studies previously described, which have all been observational, where the investigator merely observes and takes no action.

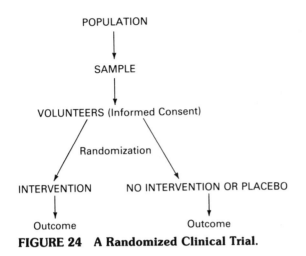

FIGURE 24   A Randomized Clinical Trial.

Informed Consent

The fact that intervention is applied to one group and withheld from another means that the participants must all be volunteers. Those asked to participate are usually at high risk for the outcome of interest (myocardial infarction, preterm delivery, or fetus with neural tube defect, for example). The request for informed consent spells out this fact, and the patient is permitted to question the interviewer administering the consent form. Regardless of whether the patient consents or declines to participate, their behavior may be modified in light of the knowledge of high-risk status and appreciation that this risk can be lowered. Despite this limitation, the randomized clinical trial yields results that cannot be obtained by any other method.

Randomization of Individuals

Random assignment to study and control groups is the procedure that will give the greatest confidence that the groups are comparable. With random allocation, the groups formed can be expected to be generally alike at the beginning of the trial. This is true for risk factors, both known and unknown. This is a crucial point to be grasped in the design of these trials. If you have two groups of patients, and you apply a different treatment to each group, you can only ascribe a difference in outcome to be the result of the differing treatment if the patients were randomized. The process of randomization is alien to the clinician, whose training and practice correctly emphasize discrimination, selection, and judgment prior to instituting treatment.

Elimination of Bias

Both investigator and participant are subjected to the influence of their respective expectations as to the efficacy of the treatment. In order to reduce bias from this source, blinding techniques are used. In double blinding, neither the subject nor the investigator knows to which group the subject is assigned. This technique is most desirable in trials where subjective endpoints, such as "improved," "unchanged," or "worse," are used. If objective endpoints, such as death or stroke, are measured, blinding is not essential.

Exercise

A randomized clinical trial, referred to as the University Group Diabetes Program (UGDP), was performed to evaluate different methods of treatment of diabetes.

The principal features of this clinical trial included the establishment of a common protocol for the collection of comparable data, random allocation of patients to treatment groups, the inclusion of a comparable placebo-treated group, double-blind evaluation of the oral drugs, long-term observation of patients, and central collection, editing, and monitoring of the study data. The patients selected for the UGDP had non-insulin dependent diabetes mellitus (NIDDM) and did not require insulin to remain symptom free. This type of diabetic constitutes the majority (over 90%) of the diabetic population.

1. **How did the selection of this type of diabetic affect the applicability of any conclusions derived from this trial?**

2. **When is double-blind evaluation most necessary? Least necessary? What does it involve?**

The UGDP had two major objectives:

a. Evaluation of the efficacy of hypoglycemic treatments in the prevention of vascular complications in a long-term, prospective, and cooperative clinical trial.
b. Study of the natural history of vascular disease in NIDDM.

The following therapy regimens were studied in the UGDP:

I. Insulin variable (IVAR): insulin is given in varying amounts in order to maintain normal blood glucose levels
II. Insulin standard (ISTD): insulin lente U-80 is given in doses ranging from 10 to 16 units per day depending on body surface
III. Tolbutamide (TOLB): 1.5 grams per day orally

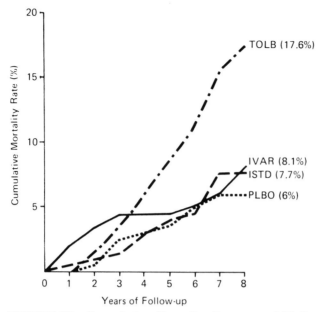

FIGURE 25 **Cumulative Mortality Rates per 100 Population at Risk by Year of Follow-Up. Cardiovascular Causes of Death Only. (Modified from Klimt et al., 1970.)**

IV. Lactose placebo (PLBO): in forms and dosage schedules corresponding to those used for the oral hypoglycemia agents

All groups received the same diet prescription.

Results

The study reached several surprising conclusions:

a. Insulin (in either dosage) is no more effective than diet alone in prolonging life among NIDDM.
b. Diet plus tolbutamide, the most commonly used oral hypoglycemic agent, is no more effective than diet alone in prolonging life in NIDDM.
c. There is a statistically significant excess of cardiovascular deaths among the tolbutamide group compared with the placebo group.

Some results are expressed in Figure 25.

3. Was it ethical to treat one group with a placebo?

4. Today it would be more difficult to carry out such a trial. Why?

5. If no placebo group had been included, which conclusions would be lost?

Beginning in 1961 patients were recruited in 12 clinical centers. The four treatment groups contained a total of 1,027 patients. All patients were assigned randomly to one of the four treatment groups.

6. **Why is randomization essential and what does it accomplish?**

Exercise Answers

1. **Any results from this study, as with any other study, are only applicable to populations similar to the study population. In this instance, however, this is not a constraint because the patients studied were representative of a large cross-section of NIDDM.**

2. **Double-blind evaluation is necessary to eliminate subjective bias by observers and subjects. It is most necessary when the outcome is subjective, such as "improved," "unchanged," or "worse." It is least necessary when an objective endpoint, such as "death," is being monitored. It involves the blind assignment of subjects to treatment and placebo groups and the blind assessment of outcome.**

3. **Informed consent was obtained from all participants, who were very closely monitored for any untoward effects. Prominent diabetologists involved in the design of the trial believed that the placebo group might fare as well as the other groups, and that belief was justified.**

4. **Today this trial may not have received clearance from an ethical viewpoint, i.e., the Human Volunteers Committee, because of the inclusion of the placebo group.**

5. **The most important conclusions would not have been reached if the placebo had been dropped, i.e., a) that insulin is not superior to placebo, and b) that tolbutamide is associated with increased risk of death due to cardiovascular causes (statistically significant) compared to the placebo.**

6. **Randomization is essential because then and only then can the difference in outcome between the groups be ascribed to the treatment applied. If randomization is omitted, the difference in outcome may be due to differing characteristics in the competing groups. Randomization achieves an unbiased distribution of risk factors (i.e., age, sex, severity of disease, etc.). This principle is the underlying concept upon which randomized clinical trials are based.**

Recommended Readings

1. Mausner, J. S., and Bahn, A. K. 1984. *Epidemiology—An Introductory Text,* second edition, chapter 7. W. B. Saunders Company, Philadelphia.
2. Lilienfeld, A. M., and Lilienfeld, D. E. 1980. *Epidemiology: Foundations,* second edition, chapter 10. Oxford University Press, New York.

Reference

Klimt, C. R., Knatterud, G. L., Meinert, C. L., and Prout, T. E. 1970. University Group Diabetes Program: A study of the effects of hypoglycemic agents on vascular complications in patients with adult onset diabetes. *Diabetes* 19 (Supp. 2):747–782.

14

Association and Causation

Objectives Covered

28. Illustrate with one example the concept of multifactorial causation of disease.
29. Define the following types of association:
a. artifactual
b. noncausal
c. causal
30. Distinguish between association and causation and list five criteria that support a causal inference.

Study Notes

Epidemiologic studies yield statistical associations between a disease and exposure. This is only the first step. We must interpret the meaning of these relationships. An association may be artifactual, noncausal, or causal.

An artifactual or spurious association may arise because of bias in the study. Sources of bias are discussed in Chapter 11. Noncausal associations occur in two ways:

1. The disease may cause the exposure (rather than the exposure causing the disease).
2. The disease and the exposure are both associated with a third factor, X, known or unknown (see Figure 26). Here, in measuring exposure we are inadvertently measuring X.

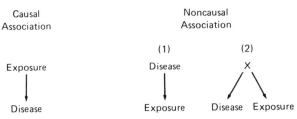

FIGURE 26 Causal and Noncausal Associations.

An example of the second type of noncausal association follows. A positive statistical association between coronary heart disease (CHD) mortality rates and coffee drinking habits has been demonstrated. Let us assume the results shown in Table 53.

TABLE 53.

Coffee Consumption (Cups per Day)	CHD Mortality in Males Ages 55–64 (Deaths per 1,000 per Year)
0	6
1–5	8
6+	12

However, it has been shown that people who drink coffee also tend to be cigarette smokers, and cigarette smoking is strongly associated with CHD mortality, as shown in Table 54.

TABLE 54.

Cigarette Consumption (Packs per Day)	CHD Mortality in Males Ages 55–64 (Deaths per 1,000 per Year)
0	4
1–2	10
3+	15

Thus, to isolate the effect of coffee drinking, we cross-clarify CHD mortality rates according to both variables (see Table 55). Examination of Table 55 reveals that when cigarette consumption is held constant, the

TABLE 55.

	CHD Mortality Rates			
Coffee		*Cigarettes (Packs per Day)*		
(Cups per Day)	0	1–2	3+	All
0	4	9	15	6
1–5	6	10	13	8
6+	5	9	16	12
All	4	10	15	

effect of coffee drinking disappears. Thus, the association between coffee drinking and CHD mortality is noncausal, mediated by cigarette smoking (Figure 27). This means that if coffee drinking is varied independently of cigarette consumption, CHD mortality rates are unchanged.

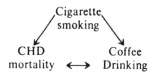

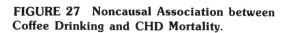

FIGURE 27 Noncausal Association between Coffee Drinking and CHD Mortality.

Multiple Causation

When an outcome is affected by multiple variables, in order to examine the influence of a single one, it is necessary to adjust for the effects of the others. An earlier example is the use of age adjustment to control for the effects of age on mortality. A simple technique for isolating a specific effect due to one variable is to examine the outcome rates, at several levels of this variable, while holding the other variables constant. This technique is cross-classification. A sophisticated approach involves the use of multiple regression analysis to measure the effect of the relative contribution of each of a series of variables on an outcome.

Medicine offers numerous examples of multiple causation. Maternal mortality, for example, is affected positively by both age and parity (number of children born). It is necessary to study women of certain parity, say 1, 2–3, 4–5, 6+, and in each of these four groups examine the relationship between age and maternal mortality. The result will be that the age effect persists in all parity groups, and the effect is very marked. If women in age groups <20, 20–29, 30–39, 40+ are classified according to parity within each of the age groups, it will be found that increasing parity exerts a small positive influence upon maternal mortality, but not nearly as marked an effect as that of age.

Causal Association

Medicine is concerned with limiting or preventing disease. The search for etiology is pursued in the hope that, once the cause of a disease is found, prevention will follow. Causality is assumed when one factor is shown to contribute to the development of disease and its removal is shown to reduce the frequency of disease. This concept of causality is different from that applied in law or philosophy. In prevention, it is sufficient to identify an exposure without necessarily identifying the ultimate cause of the disease. For example, cigarette smoke has been identified as the contaminated substance that is associated with increased rates of lung and other cancers and heart and respiratory diseases. It is unnecessary to identify precisely which component in the smoke is the prime offender before instituting preventive measures.

Establishing Causation

Statistical methods alone cannot establish proof of a causal relationship in an association. Interpretation of such an association must be conducted in a systematic manner (see Figure 28).

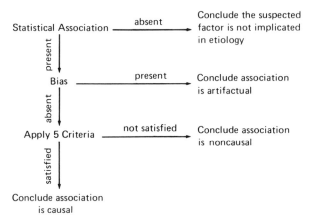

FIGURE 28   Interpretation of Results of an Epidemiological Study.

The advisory committee to the Surgeon General of the Public Health Service (Advisory Committee, 1964) defined five criteria that should be fulfilled to establish a causal relationship. These five criteria have been generally adopted as a test of causation. They are:

1. the consistency of the association
2. the strength of the association
3. the specificity of the association
4. the temporal relationship of the association
5. the coherence of the association

The definitions are summarized below:

1. Consistency means that different studies resulted in the same association, despite the fact that they employed different designs and were conducted on different populations, sometimes in different countries.
2. Strength refers to the size of the relative risk found. The greater the relative risk, the more convincing it is that the association is causal. Furthermore, if a dose-response gradient can be demonstrated, the likelihood that the exposure is causal increases. Such dose-response gradients may be recorded as the degree (the number of cigarettes smoked daily, for example) or duration of exposure (the length of time for which oral contraceptives have been used).

3. Specificity measures the degree to which one particular exposure produces one specific disease. If the biological response to the exposure is variable, it is less likely to be causal.
4. Temporal relationship means exposure to the factor must precede development of the disease.
5. Coherence means biological plausibility, which may have been established in animal models.

The five criteria quoted above are the best guide to etiology in the absence of a controlled experiment, but they cannot be considered to be a substitute for the latter.

Exercise

1. **Table 56a–c gives the results of a study of the factors associated with response to a cervical cancer screening program.**

TABLE 56a. Response to Program by Social Class

Social Class	Percent Population Responding
High social class	75
Low social class	46
All social classes	53

TABLE 56b. Response to Program by Marital Status

Marital Status	Percent Population Responding
Married	82
Single	68
Widowed and divorced	43
All marital status	53

TABLE 56c. Percent of Persons in Each Subgroup (Social Class by Marital Status) Responding to Program

Social Class	Married	Single	Widowed and/or Divorced	All Marital Status
High social class	83	67	43	75
Low social class	81	69	43	46
All social classes	82	68	43	53

From these data it would be correct to infer that:
a. Married women respond better.
b. No inferences can be drawn from these tables because the

marital status of high and low social class people is not
shown.

c. Married people have a higher response rate than do the single or widowed because more of them are in a high social class.

d. No inference can be drawn from these tables because it is not known if this is a cohort or case-control study.

2. Table 57 shows the data obtained in a cross-sectional study of obesity and blood pressure.

TABLE 57.   Relationship of Obesity to Level of Blood Pressure (Expressed as Numbers of People)

	Low Blood Pressure	Intermediate Blood Pressure	High Blood Pressure	Total
Obese	50	50	100	200
Normal weight	170	30	100	300
Thin (nonobese)	380	20	100	500
Total	600	100	300	1000

From these data, which of the following conclusions may be correct:

a. 50/100 = 50% of those with intermediate blood pressure are obese.

b. 100/1000 = 10% of those with high blood pressure are obese.

c. 50/200 = 25% of the obese have low blood pressure.

d. 100/500 = 20% of those with high blood pressure are thin.

3. The association between cigarette smoking and lung cancer has been subjected to considerable scrutiny. Which of the following statements both strengthen the association between cigarette smoking and lung cancer and move the evidence towards the direction of a causal relationship?

a. The risk of lung cancer increases as the daily consumption of cigarettes increases and/or as the duration of smoking lengthens.

b. Ex-smokers have lung cancer incidence rates intermediate between those of nonsmokers and current smokers.

c. Animal experiments have shown an increased incidence of precancerous lesions following tobacco smoke inhalation.

d. Prospective studies agree with retrospective studies about the presence and direction of the association.

4. Retrospective studies have shown a higher level of stress in the year prior to a heart attack as reported by survivors than reported by controls. Can it can concluded from this study that stress causes heart attacks?

5. Cross-sectional studies (surveys) reveal that a higher proportion of Arizona residents have respiratory diseases than residents of other states. Can it be concluded from this that living in Arizona causes respiratory disease?

6. A study of stillbirths and congenital malformations revealed that a higher proportion of mothers of such children had taken steroids during pregnancy than a control group of mothers of normal children. From this information, may we conclude that taking steroids during pregnancy causes stillbirths and congenital malformations?

Exercise Answers

1. a. Married women respond better regardless of social class. Table 56a seems to indicate that the response is associated with social class. Table 56b seems to indicate that the response is associated with marital status. However, Table 56c reveals that if social class is held constant, the influence of marital status persists, but that if marital status is held constant, the influence of social class disappears.

2. a and c are correct.

3. a, b, c, and d are all correct.

4. No. It is unclear if stress caused the heart attack or if the heart attack caused the stress or some other unknown factor caused both. The question must be examined prospectively.

5. Not necessarily. Those with respiratory disease may have migrated to Arizona because of the climate.

6. Not necessarily. The difficulty with such studies is that the steroids may have been prescribed because of a history of bleeding or contractions during pregnancy or for mothers with a poor obstetric history. The association may be noncausal.

Recommended Readings

1. Mausner, J. S., and Bahn, A. K. 1984. *Epidemiology—An Introductory Text,* second edition, chapter 8. W. B. Saunders Company, Philadelphia.

2. Lilienfeld, A. M., and Lilienfeld, D. E. 1980. *Epidemiology: Foundations,* second edition, chapter 12. Oxford University Press, New York.

Reference

Advisory Committee to the Surgeon General of the Public Health Service. 1964. *Smoking and Health.* P.H.S. Publication No. 1103, pp. 182–189. Public Health Service, Washington, D.C.

Self-Assessment 3

Objectives Covered: 25–30

Best Choice—Select *One* Answer Only

46. In a cross-sectional study of peptic ulcer in a community, persons meeting the symptomatic criteria for peptic ulcer were found in 80 per 100,000 men ages 35–49 and 90 per 100,000 women ages 35–49. The inference that in this age group, women are at a greater risk of developing peptic ulcer is:
    a. correct
    b. incorrect due to failure to distinguish between incidence and prevalence
    c. incorrect because rates were used to compare males and females
    d. incorrect due to failure to recognize a possible cohort effect
    e. incorrect because there is no comparison or control group

47. Epidemiologic studies of the roles of a suspected factor in the etiology of a disease may be observational or experimental. The essential difference between experimental and observational studies is that in experimental investigations:
    a. The study and control groups are equal in size.
    b. The study is prospective.
    c. The study and control groups are always compatible.
    d. The investigator determines who shall be exposed to the suspected factor and who shall not.
    e. Controls are used.

48. Which of the following factors is the most important to the validity of the conclusions drawn from a clinical trial?
    a. equal numbers of treated and placebo individuals
    b. follow-up of 100% of the participants
    c. effective randomization of participants
    d. a relatively high incidence of the disease in the population studied
    e. inclusion in both groups of individuals of all ages

49. In a prospective study of a disease, the cohort originally selected consisted of:
    a. persons who are found to have the disease
    b. persons without the disease
    c. persons with the factor under investigation
    d. persons with a family history of the disease
    e. persons without the factor under investigation

50. Table 58 shows the results from a study of the determinants of juvenile delinquency.
    What would you conclude from these results?
    a. Broken homes seem to be a cause of juvenile delinquency.
    b. Both broken homes and high SES independently are causes of juvenile delinquency.

TABLE 58.

	Percent Delinquency According to Type of Home	P
Children from broken homes	14	<0.05
Children from intact homes	5	
	Percent Delinquency According to Socioeconomic Status of Family	
Children from high SES	16	<0.05
Children from low SES	4	

    c. The effect of broken homes should be examined with each socioeconomic class.
    d. Neither of the above statements can be made because the proportions are too small.
    e. Socioeconomic status determines both broken homes and juvenile delinquency.

51. A "double blind" study of a vaccine is one in which:
    a. The study group receives the vaccine and the control group receives a placebo.
    b. Neither observer nor subjects know the nature of the placebo.
    c. Neither observer nor subjects know which subject receives the vaccine and which receives a placebo.
    d. Neither the study group nor the control group knows the identity of the observers.
    e. The control group does not know the identity of the study group.

52. A major weakness of retrospective studies of the role of a suspected factor in the etiology of a disease, as compared with prospective studies, is that:
    a. They are more costly and take longer.
    b. There may be bias in determining the presence or absence of the suspected factor.
    c. There may be bias in determining the presence or absence of the resulting disease.
    d. It is more difficult to obtain controls.
    e. It is more difficult to assure comparability of cases and controls.

53. A cohort must have:
    a. same year of birth
    b. passage through the same time period
    c. common place of residence
    d. exposure to the same disease
    e. common disease history

54. At the initial examination in the Framingham study, coronary heart disease was found in 5 per 1,000 men ages 30–44 and in 5 per 1,000 women ages 30–44. The inference that in this age group men and women have an equal risk of developing coronary heart disease is:
    a. correct
    b. incorrect because of failure to distinguish between incidence and prevalence

   c. incorrect because a proportionate ratio is used when a rate is required to support the inference
   d. incorrect because of failure to recognize a possible cohort phenomenon
   e. incorrect because there is no control or comparison group
55. Which of the following is an advantage of a retrospective study?
   a. There is little or no bias in assessment of exposure to the factor.
   b. Multiple disease outcomes following a selected exposure can be readily studied.
   c. Dependence on recall by subjects in the study is minimized.
   d. It is possible to determine the true incidence rate of the disease.
   e. It may be used to study etiology of a rare disease.
56. An orthopedic surgeon published the data relating to the management of 204 patients, who sustained fractures of the femoral neck. Table 59 gives mortality data relating to patients who were treated surgically (by open reduction with pinning) or conservatively (by closed reduction with immobilization).

TABLE 59.

	Surgical Treatments	Conservative Management	Total
Number of:			
Patients	139	65	204
Survivors	103	34	137
Deaths	36	31	67
Percent mortality	26.5%	47.7%	32.9%
$\chi^2 = 8.57; P < 0.01$			

The most reasonable interpretation of the data is:
   a. The statistically significant decrease noted in the mortality rate of the patients who underwent surgery means that surgery is the treatment of choice in fractures of the femoral neck.
   b. The unusually large number of patients in the surgical group distorts the results.
   c. No interpretation is possible because information is lacking on the residual functional disability of patients in both groups.
   d. Patients being managed conservatively may be older and sicker than those selected for surgery.
   e. The data are useless in that deaths subsequent to discharge are not given.
57. In 1945, 1,000 women were identified who worked in a factory painting radium dials on watches. The incidence of bone cancer in these women up to 1975 was compared to that of 1,000 women who worked as telephone operators in 1945. Twenty of the radium dial painters and four of the telephone operators developed bone cancer between 1945 and 1975. This study is an example of a:
   a. prospective study
   b. experimental study
   c. clinical trial
   d. cross-sectional study
   e. retrospective study
58. A common medical belief states that after a certain surgical operation it is dangerous for women to have children. An interested physician studied the

records of a group of women who had survived this operation. For each woman the records showed the number of children born and the number of years the women lived after the operation. The physician observed that on the average the more children a woman bore after the operation the longer she lived. He concluded the traditional medical belief was a fallacy. This conclusion is incorrect because:

a. The doctor's sample was biased since it included only survivors of the operation.
b. The longer a woman lives after the operation, the more children she is likely to have.
c. The doctor should have concluded that the traditional belief is correct.
d. The older women in the group were probably past childbearing age.
e. The older women probably did not survive the operation.

59. The following vaccine trial was performed: 1,000 randomly selected children two years of age were given a vaccine against a certain disease and followed for 10 years. Of these, 80% were never afflicted with the disease. Which is the most correct conclusion regarding the efficacy of the vaccine?

a. The vaccine is an excellent one because of the high rate of immunization.
b. No conclusion is possible since no follow-up was made of nonvaccinated children.
c. The vaccine is not very effective because it should have produced a higher immunization rate.
d. No conclusion is possible since no test of statistical significance was performed.
e. The significant figure is $100\% - 80\% = 20\%$, the rate of acquiring the illness.

60. In a study designed to measure the frequency of minor symptoms due to administration of a drug:

a. Control subjects who receive no medication are necessary in order to interpret the data.
b. Control subjects who receive a placebo are necessary in order to interpret the data.
c. The inclusion of controls is apt to mislead the investigator, especially if the incidence of adverse reaction is low.
d. The desirability of having controls depends on the kind of reactions expected.
e. The desirability of having controls depends on the ages of the subjects.

61. The data from a study of age versus prevalence of obesity are shown in Table 60.

TABLE 60.

Age	Percent Obese
10–40	19
40–60	25
60–80	15
80+	5

The inference that as people grow older, they become thinner is:

a. correct
b. incorrect because a rate is necessary to support the observation

   c. incorrect because no control or comparison group is used
   d. incorrect because no such conclusion should be made from cross-sectional data
   e. incorrect because prevalence is used whereas incidence is necessary
62. Which of the following is a retrospective study?
   a. Study of previous mortality and/or morbidity trends to permit estimates of the occurrence of disease in the future.
   b. Analysis of previous research in different places and under different circumstances to permit establishment of a hypothesis based on cumulative knowledge of all known factors identified in the disease under study.
   c. Obtaining histories and other information from a group of known cases and from a comparison group to determine the relative frequency of characteristics under study in cases.
   d. Study of relative risk of cancer among men who have quit and controls who still smoke.
   e. A survey of the prevalence of a disease in the different strata of a population.

K-type Questions

Key

a	b	c	d	e
1, 2, 3	1 and 3	2 and 4	only 4	all 4
are correct	are correct	are correct	is correct	are correct

63. "Matching" is undertaken in a case-control study so that:
   1. Variables already known to influence the distribution of the disease under study are controlled for in both case and comparison groups.
   2. The influence of the variables matched for may be studied.
   3. The result may not be attributed to the influence of the matched variables.
   4. The study results may include inferences about the influence of the preselected matching variables.
64. To be causally related to a disease, an etiological factor must satisfy the following conditions:
   1. The factor is found more frequently among the diseased than the nondiseased.
   2. Exposure to the factor must precede the development of the disease.
   3. Elimination of the factor reduces the risk of the disease.
   4. The factor is found among all cases with the disease.
65. Controls are needed in a case-control retrospective study because:
   1. They are matched to the cases for suspected etiological factors.
   2. They may be followed to determine if they develop the disease in question.
   3. They increase the sample size, so that statistical significance may be achieved.
   4. They allow evaluation of whether or not the frequency of a characteristic or past exposure among the cases is different from that among comparable persons in the population who are free of the disease.

Self-Assessment Final

Objectives Covered: 1–30

Best Choice—Select *One* Answer Only

66. The number of new cancer cases (per 100,000 population) per year for selected sites occurring in men ages 55–59 in two populations is shown on Table 61.

TABLE 61.

	Number of New Cases per 100,000 Men per Year	
	Population A	*Population B*
Lung	40	55
Colon and rectum	20	30
Prostate	12	15

The inference that men ages 55–59 in population B are more prone to cancer of the lung, colon and rectum, and prostate than are men ages 55–59 in population A is:
a. correct
b. incorrect because of failure to distinguish between incidence and prevalence
c. incorrect because proportionate mortality alone does not give an estimate of risk
d. incorrect because of failure to adjust for differences in the age structure of the two populations
e. incorrect because there is no control or comparison group

67. In the investigation of an epidemic of food poisoning at a banquet, high attack rates were found for people who ate roast beef as well as those who ate mushroom sauce. Table 62 shows combinations of the two foods that were then considered.

TABLE 62.

	Ate Mushroom Sauce			Did Not Eat Mushroom Sauce		
	Number	*Number Ill*	*Attack Rate (%)*	*Number*	*Number Ill*	*Attack Rate (%)*
Ate roast beef	150	105	70	72	2	3
Did not eat roast beef	42	33	78	26	0	0

Thus, the infective item is most likely to be:
a. mushroom sauce
b. roast beef
c. the combination of roast beef with mushroom sauce
d. mushroom sauce without roast beef
e. neither roast beef nor mushroom sauce

68. In an advertisement for raspberry-flavored aureomycin it was claimed that, "Out of 1,000 children with upper respiratory infection treated with our raspberry flavored aureomycin, 970 were asymptomatic within 72 hours." The inference that in a child with upper respiratory infection, raspberry-flavored aureomycin is the treatment of choice is:
a. correct
b. incorrect because the comparison is not based on rates
c. incorrect because no control or comparison group is used
d. incorrect because no test of statistical significance is made
e. incorrect because a cohort effect may be operating

69. A study covering records of 300 deaths in white children from accidental poisoning reported in City A showed that among those who died, there were five times as many children whose socioeconomic conditions were rated as low than there were children whose socioeconomic conditions were rated as high. The inference that accidental poisoning is five times more common among children from families of low socioeconomic status than among those of high socioeconomic status in City A is:
a. correct
b. incorrect because the study and comparison groups are not comparable or relevant
c. incorrect because there is improper interpretation of statistical significance
d. incorrect because the comparison is not based on rates
e. incorrect because observer or interviewer bias may account for the results

70. Community A and Community B each have crude mortality rates for coronary heart disease (CHD) of 4 per 1,000. The age-adjusted CHD mortality rate is 5 per 1,000 for Community A and 3 per 1,000 for Community B. One may conclude that:
a. Community A has a younger population than Community B.
b. Community A has an older population than Community B.
c. The two communities have identical age distribution.
d. Diagnosis is more accurate in Community A than in Community B.
e. Diagnosis is less accurate in Community A than in Community B.

71. A retrospective study is characterized by all except the following:
a. It is relatively inexpensive.
b. Relative risk may be estimated from the results.
c. Incidence rates may be computed.
d. One selects controls without the disease.
e. Assessment of past exposure may be biased.

72. The risk of acquiring a disease is measured by the:
a. incidence rate
b. incidence rate times the average duration of the disease
c. incidence rate divided by the prevalence rate
d. prevalence rate
e. prevalence rate times the average duration of the disease

73. A study of traffic safety in Minnesota showed that 61% of those involved in accidents last year had more than 10 years of driving experience, 21% had 6 to 10 years experience, and 17% had 1 to 5 years. Traffic experts concluded that experience seems to make drivers more complacent and careless. Which of the following best states why this conclusion is not justified?
    a. The rates have not been standardized for age differences.
    b. The data are incomplete because of unreported accidents.
    c. A comparison needs to be made with similar data on drivers not involved in accidents.
    d. No test of statistical significance has been made.
    e. Prevalence is used where incidence is required.

74. The strength of an association between a factor and a disease is best measured by:
    a. incubation period
    b. incidence of the disease in the total population
    c. prevalence of the factor
    d. attributable risk
    e. relative risk

75. Table 63 shows the relative frequency of newly reported cancers of specific sites in two populations.

TABLE 63.

Site of Cancer	Percent of Total	
	Population A	Population B
Lung	10.0	6.7
Breast	30.0	20.0
Uterus	25.0	16.7
All other	35.0	56.6
Total: all sites	100.0	100.0

The inference that population A seems to be more prone to cancer of the lung, breast, and uterus than is population B is:
    a. correct
    b. incorrect because of failure to distinguish between incidence and prevalence
    c. incorrect because a proportionate ratio is used when a rate is required to support the inference
    d. incorrect because of failure to recognize a possible cohort phenomenon
    e. incorrect because there is no control or comparison group

76. An investigation of an outbreak of diarrhea revealed that the proportion of cases eating in Restaurant A was 85%, Restaurant B was 15%, Restaurant C was 55%, and the proportion consuming public water was 95%. Which of the following statements is correct?
    a. The source is Restaurant A because it has the highest proportion of cases among the restaurants.
    b. The source is not Restaurant B because it has the lowest rate.

    c. The source is the water supply because it has the highest proportion of cases.

    d. The source could be either Restaurant A, Restaurant C, or the water supply.

    e. Similar data on a well group must be collected to reach a valid conclusion.

77. "Case fatality rate" for a given disease refers to:

    a. the crude death rate per 100,000 population

    b. cause-specific death rate due to the disease

    c. a fatal outcome of any disease

    d. the percentage of deaths among cases of the disease

    e. the proportion of deaths due to the disease among all deaths from all causes

78. An investigator is interested in the etiology of neonatal jaundice. To study this condition, he selected 100 children who were diagnosed with this condition and 100 children born in the same time period and in the same hospital who did not have a diagnosis of neonatal jaundice. He then reviewed the obstetric and delivery records of their mothers to determine various prenatal and perinatal exposures. This is an example of a:

    a. cross-sectional study

    b. retrospective study

    c. prospective study

    d. clinical trial

    e. an experiment

79. A study of all women ages 20–25 years old in a large industrial state found that the annual rate of new cases of cervical cancer in women who used oral contraceptives was 5/100,000 and that it was 2/100,000 in those who did not use oral contraceptives. On the basis of these data, the inference that taking oral contraceptives causes cervical cancer is:

    a. correct

    b. incorrect due to failure to distinguish between incidence and prevalence

    c. incorrect due to failure to adjust for possible differences in age distributions of users and nonusers

    d. incorrect because a proportion is used when a rate is required to support the inference

    e. incorrect because the two groups may differ in other relevant factors

80. Which of the following statements describes the major advantages of a randomized clinical trial?

    a. It avoids observer bias.

    b. It lends itself to ethical justification.

    c. It yields results replicable in other patients.

    d. It rules out self-selection of participants to the different treatment groups.

    e. It enrolls representative patients.

81. A survey conducted in England revealed that of 224 families in which there had been a known case of poliomyelitis, 56 maintained parakeets as a family pet. In another British survey, 30 of 99 poliomyelitis patients questioned kept parakeets. The inference that there is some relationship between the presence of a parakeet in a household and the occurrence of poliomyelitis among household members is:

    a. correct

    b. incorrect because of failure to distinguish between incidence and prevalence

    c. incorrect because a proportionate ratio is used when a rate is required to support the inference

    d. incorrect because of failure to recognize a possible cohort phenomenon

    e. incorrect because there is no control or comparison group

82. A controversy occurred between the proponents of drug therapy and remedial reading for patients with dyslexia. To support their position, one party wrote, "Of 119 patients with dyslexia, 97 showed improvement following remedial reading courses." The inference that in patients with dyslexia, remedial reading is the therapy of choice is:

    a. correct

    b. incorrect because the comparison is not based on rates

    c. incorrect because no control or comparison group is being used

    d. incorrect because no test of statistical significance is being made

    e. incorrect because a cohort effect may be operating

83. An investigator determines the correlation coefficient between triglyceride levels and degree of atherosclerosis in sampled blood vessels to be $+1.67$. On the basis of this you would conclude that:

    a. Triglyceride level is a good predictor of atherosclerosis.

    b. Triglyceride level is not a good predictor of atherosclerosis.

    c. High triglyceride levels cause atherosclerosis.

    d. Atherosclerosis causes high triglyceride levels.

    e. The investigator has incorrectly determined the correlation coefficient.

Table 64 describes the survival of cancer patients following a new drug treatment.

TABLE 64.

Interval	Patient Alive at Beginning of Interval	Patients Who Died during Interval	Proportion of Those Alive at Beginning of Interval Who Died During Interval
0–3 months	1,000	300	0.3
3–6 months	700	140	0.2
6–12 months	560	112	0.2
12–18 months	448	224	0.5
18–24 months	224	90	0.4

Use these data for questions 84–86.

84. The probability that a patient survives for two years after the treatment, given that they have survived for six months, is:

    a. $134/560 = 0.24$

    b. $426/560 = 0.76$

    c. $134/700 = 0.19$

    d. $426/700 = 0.61$

    e. cannot be determined from these data

85. The probability that a patient survives for three months after the treatment began is:

    a. 0.3

    b. 0.4
    c. 0.5
    d. 0.6
    e. 0.7

86. The probability that a patient dies within two years after the treatment is:
    a. $90/224 = 0.4$
    b. $866/1000 = 0.866$
    c. $90/1000 = 0.09$
    d. $224/1000 = 0.224$
    e. cannot be determined from these data

87. A study was conducted to assess a new surgical procedure designed to reduce the incidence of postoperative complications. The incidence of complications was found to be 40% in 25 patients having the new procedure and 60% for 20 patients having the old procedure. This difference is not statistically significant. Thus, it may be concluded that:
    a. The new procedure is effective in reducing postoperative complications.
    b. The new procedure is ineffective in reducing postoperative complications.
    c. The sample is biased.
    d. The result is clinically significant.
    e. The evidence is insufficient to demonstrate that the new procedure is effective in reducing postoperative complications.

88. A screening test of known sensitivity and specificity is applied to two populations. The prevalence of the disease being screened for is 10% in population A and 1% in population B. Which of the following is true?
    a. The percent of all negative tests that are false negatives is lower in population A than in population B.
    b. Specificity is lower in population A than in population B.
    c. Reliability is higher in population A than in population B.
    d. The percent of all positive tests that are false positives is lower in population A than in population B.
    e. Sensitivity is higher in population A than in population B.

89. Two plans for the follow-up treatment of newly detected hypertensives were tried in a community. Plan A was used in the eastern and southern districts of the community while Plan B was used in the northern and western districts. Table 65 shows the data obtained three years after the start of these plans.

TABLE 65.

	Plan A	Plan B
Number of hypertensives	2,200	1,900
Percent of hypertensives successfully treated	41	45

The differences in success rates for the two plans were statistically significant ($P < 0.01$). Health officials, however, decided not to change to Plan B in the eastern and southern districts because the magnitude of the difference was so small. This implies that:
    a. They attributed the difference in success rates to chance alone.
    b. They felt the samples were too small to justify a decision in favor of Plan B.
    c. They felt the P value was too small to justify a decision in favor of Plan B.

d. They distinguished between statistical significance and practical importance of the difference in success rates.

e. They felt that the success rates should be higher than 50 percent.

K-type Questions

Key

a	b	c	d	e
1, 2, 3	1 and 3	2 and 4	only 4	all 4
are correct	are correct	are correct	is correct	are correct

90. The I.Q.'s of a class of students are distributed according to the normal curve, with a mean of 115 and a standard deviation of 10. This means that:
   1. 50% will have I.Q.'s less than 115.
   2. 5% will have I.Q.'s less than 105.
   3. 2.5% will have I.Q.'s greater than 135.
   4. 2.5% will have I.Q.'s greater than 125.

91. To determine attack rates for a respiratory disease of unknown origin among people attending an American Legion Convention in Philadelphia, random samples of guests staying at four hotels were surveyed for subsequent illness. Since it was not feasible to survey all the guests, random sampling provided the best information because:
   1. It would identify all cases of the disease.
   2. It would avoid biases introduced by the method of selecting guests for study.
   3. It would eliminate sampling error.
   4. It would give each guest an equal chance of being selected.

92. A series of 1,000 female patients with breast cancer contained 32 who were pregnant. From this, one may conclude:
   1. Pregnancy is a rare complication of breast cancer.
   2. If age adjustments are made we can determine the risk of breast cancer during pregnancy.
   3. Breast cancer is a rare complication of pregnancy.
   4. In this series 3.2% of the breast cancer patients were pregnant.

93. In a study to determine whether or not tonsillectomy is associated with subsequent development of Hodgkin's disease, the estimated relative risk of developing the disease for those with a prior tonsillectomy was found to be 2.9. From this we may conclude:
   1. The case fatality rate is higher among those with a prior tonsillectomy.
   2. The rate of Hodgkin's disease cases is higher among those with a prior tonsillectomy.
   3. Tonsillectomy appears to protect against the development of Hodgkin's disease.
   4. The incidence of Hodgkin's disease among those with a prior tonsillectomy is 2.9 times that of those with intact tonsils.

94. Correct statements concerning retrospective and prospective studies include:
   1. Prospective studies are likely to be less susceptible to bias.
   2. Prospective studies permit direct determination of incidence rates.
   3. The retrospective approach has the advantage that data are readily at hand for quick analysis.

    4. The prospective approach is often used to elucidate factors related to rare diseases.
95. Table 66 shows the incidence of retrolentalfibroplasia (RLF) by sex of the infant at the Boston Lying-In Hospital, 1938–52.

TABLE 66.

	Number of Premature Infants	RLF Cases	RLF Percent
Males	260	45	17.3
Females	321	54	16.8

The chi-square value was found to be 0.02 and the P value was greater than 0.10. The implication of this result is that:
1. The sex of the infant is probably not a determinant of RLF.
2. It is probable that the difference in incidence of RLF between the sexes can be explained by chance alone.
3. The difference in incidence of RLF between the sexes is not statistically significant.
4. RLF is probably associated with sex of the infant.

96. In general, screening should be undertaken for diseases with the following features:
1. disease for which there is an effective primary prevention measure available
2. disease with a high prevalence in distinct segments of the population
3. diseases that are readily diagnosed and no treatment is available
4. diseases with a natural history that can be altered by medical intervention

97. Table 67 shows the data from a comparison of mortality rates due to cancer of the uterus in users and nonusers of supplemental estrogen.

TABLE 67.

	Mortality Rates (per 100,000) Age 40–54	Mortality Rates (per 100,000) Age 55–70
Users of estrogen	3.0	17.0
Nonusers	1.0	6.0

Valid conclusions derived from the above data concerning mortality among estrogen users include:
1. The mortality rates for cancer of the uterus are higher in estrogen users in both age groups studied.
2. A causal relationship is demonstrated between the use of estrogen and incidence of uterine cancer.
3. Mortality from cancer of the uterus rises with age regardless of whether or not estrogen is used.
4. The mortality rate is lower in nonusers than users because the symptoms of uterine cancer are detected earlier in the former group of women.

98. Data for patients at a certain hospital show the mean length of stay is 10 days

and the median is eight days. The most frequent length of stay is six days. From these facts we conclude:

1. Approximately 50% of the patients stay less than six days.
2. The distribution of length of stay is not symmetric.
3. The standard deviation is two days.
4. The mean length of stay is affected by stays of very long duration.

99. A random sample of teenage prenatal patients seen at University Hospital during 1973 had a mean hematocrit of 29 with a standard error of 1.5. From this information we may conclude that:

   1. The normal range for hematocrit among teenage prenatal patients is 26 to 32.
   2. It is to be expected that 95% of all teenage prenatal patients will have hematocrit levels between 26 and 32.
   3. The range 26 to 32 will include 95% of all teenage prenatal patients seen at University Hospital in 1973.
   4. The range 26 to 32 will include the mean of all teenage prenatal patients seen at University Hospital in 1973 with 95% probability.

100. The median survival time of children with leukemia treated with a combination of drugs and radiation is reported to be 28.2 months. This implies that:

   1. A child with leukemia treated with a combination of drugs and radiation can be expected to survive 56.4 months.
   2. Half of the children with leukemia treated with a combination of drugs and radiation survive more than 28.2 months.
   3. None of the children with leukemia treated with a combination of drugs and radiation survive beyond 56.4 months.
   4. Half of the children with leukemia treated with a combination of drugs and radiation survive less than 28.2 months.

Answers to Self-Assessments

1. b	26. b	51. c	76. e
2. b	27. c	52. b	77. d
3. b	28. a	53. b	78. b
4. e	29. b	54. b	79. e
5. c	30. d	55. e	80. d
6. c	31. c	56. d	81. e
7. c	32. c	57. a	82. c
8. c	33. c	58. b	83. e
9. c	34. a	59. b	84. a
10. b	35. d	60. b	85. e
11. a	36. d	61. d	86. b
12. e	37. c	62. c	87. e
13. e	38. c	63. b	88. d
14. e	39. d	64. a	89. d
15. c	40. a	65. d	90. b
16. b	41. c	66. a	91. c
17. d	42. b	67. a	92. d
18. a	43. c	68. c	93. c
19. d	44. d	69. d	94. a
20. c	45. a	70. a	95. a
21. a	46. b	71. c	96. c
22. b	47. d	72. a	97. b
23. c	48. c	73. c	98. c
24. e	49. b	74. e	99. d
25. c	50. c	75. c	100. c

Index

A

Absolute risk, 33
Age, and mortality, 20
Age-adjusted death rates, 20–21
Age-specific death rates, 20
Association, 117
  artifactual, 117
  causal, 119
  noncausal, 117
Attack rate, 2–3
  calculated by age, 8–9
Attributable risk, 33–35
  defined, 33

B

Bias, 97–98
  avoiding, by use of prospective
    studies, 104
  elimination of, in randomized
    trials, 113

C

Case-control studies, 95–101
Case fatality rates, 22
Causation
  establishing, 120–121
    criteria for, 120
  multiple, 119
Cause-specific death rates, 22
Central tendency, indices of, 45–46
Chi-square, 75–76
Coherence, defined, 121

Cohort, 103, 107
  defined, 107
  use of, in prospective studies, 103
Cohort effect, 107
Cohort studies, 103
Common-source outbreak, 3, 4
Complex events, 54
Conditional probability, 53–54
Confidence limits, 68
Consistency, defined, 120
Correlation coefficient, 81–85
Cross-sectional studies, 107–108
Crude death rate, 19–20
  defined, 19
Crude mortality rate, see Crude
    death rate
Cumulative frequency plot, 45, 47

D

Death rate
  and age, 20
  age-adjusted, 20–21
  age-specific, 20
  cause-specific, 22
  crude, 19–20
  race-specific, 21–22
  sex-specific, 21
Dependent variable, 81
Disease
  cases, classifications of, 3
  etiology, sequence of investigation
    for, 96

Distribution, *see* Frequency distribution

E
Epidemic
  characteristics, 7–9
    of person, 7
    of place, 8
    of time, 7
  defined, 3
  investigation of, 3, 7 ff.
Epidemic curve, 3–4
Epidemiology
  compared to clinical medicine, 1
  defined, 1
Experimental studies
  defined, 95
  see also Randomized clinical trial
Exposure rates, calculation of, 5, 96

F
False negatives, 62
False positives, 62
Frequency distribution, 43–45
  defined, 43
  normal curve, 46–47
  skewed, 45, 46
  symmetric, 45, 46

G
Gaussian distribution, 46

H
Histogram, 44
Hypothesis, testing, 74

I
Incidence, 27–29, 103
  defined, 27
Independent events, 53
Independent variable, 81
Informed consent, 112

L
Least squares, 82
Longitudinal, defined, 109

M
Matching, 98
Mean, defined, 45
Median, defined, 45
Mode, defined, 45
Mortality
  and age, 20
  proportionate mortality ratio, 23
  see also Death rate
Mutually exclusive events, 54

N
Normal distribution curve, 46
Normal limits, 47
Normal range, 47
Null hypothesis, 74

O
Observational studies, 95
Odds ratio, 100–101

P
P value, 74–75
Percentile defined, 45
PMR, *see* Proportionate mortality ratio
Predictive value, 62
Prevalence, 27–29
  defined, 27
  determining, 107
Probabilities, combining
  addition rule, 55
  multiplication rule, 54–55
Probability
  conditional, 53–54
  defined, 53
Proportionate mortality ratio, 23
Prospective, defined, 103
Prospective studies
  advantages and disadvantages of, 106
  analysis of results, 105–106

Prospective studies (*cont.*)
  computation of relative risk from,
    106
  defined, 103
  described, 103–107
  persons lost to follow-up, 105
  use of employed groups in, 104

R
Race-specific death rates, 21–22
Randomization, 112
Randomized clinical trial, described,
  111–113
Random sampling, 68
Range
  defined, 46
  normal, 47
Rate, 1–2
  computation of, 1
Regression equation, 82
Relative risk, 33–35
  defined, 33
  estimating from retrospective
    study, 101
Retrospective, defined, 103
Retrospective studies
  advantages and disadvantages of,
    106
  defined, 96
  described, 96–99
Risk
  absolute, 33–35
  attributable, 33–35
  relative, 33–35

S
Sample size, 75
Sampling
  bias, 67
  confidence limits, 68
  random, 68
  target population for, 67
Sampling error, 67–68

Scattergram, 81–82
Screening
  defined, 59
  tests
    acceptability, 63
    false positives and negatives, 62
    predictive value, 62
    sensitivity of, 59–61
    specificity of, 59–61
Sensitivity, 59–61
Sex-specific death rates, 21–22
Significance level, 74
Skewed distribution, 45, 46
Specificity, 59–61
Standard deviation, defined, 46
Standard error, 68
Statistical significance
  compared to clinical significance,
    75
  defined, 74
  tests for, 74
Statistical test, 73–74
Strength of association, defined,
    120
Studies
  case-control, 96–99
  cohort, 103–107
  cross-sectional, 107–108
  experimental and observational,
    95
  prospective, 103–107
  retrospective, 96–99
Symmetric distribution, 45, 46

T
Target population, defined, 67
Temporal relationship, defined, 121

V
Variable
  dependent, 81
  independent, 81
Variation, indices of, 46